Surrealism and Psychoanalysis in Grace Pailthorpe's Life and Work

This book outlines the life and intellectual thought of the English surrealist artist and psychoanalyst, Dr Grace Pailthorpe (1883–1971). It gathers her published and unpublished writings, providing an in-depth study of the importance of Surrealism in her work and legacy.

Pailthorpe's theoretical understanding of the psyche informed her approach to art, setting her work apart from other Surrealist artists by unifying artistic, scientific, and therapeutic aims. Pailthorpe considered Surrealism to be a method of investigation into unconscious mental life and believed that it was essential that the repressed part of our minds should find expression. Her theories were influenced by personal and professional experiences such as her work with female offenders, her psychoanalytic training, and her research project with Reuben Mednikoff. By bringing her artistic and theoretical work to light, Montanaro and Stefana reassert Pailthorpe's significance to the histories of both psychoanalysis and Surrealism, rendering the cross-disciplinary relevance of her work accessible to a contemporary audience.

This book is a rich resource for scholars and students interested in psychoanalysis and art history and provides an invaluable case study for the continuing significance of visual artistic practices to clinical work.

Lee Ann Montanaro, PhD, is a university lecturer and researcher. She specialises in twentieth-century literature and art. Her research interests include Surrealism, psychoanalysis, modernism, and comparative literature.

Alberto Stefana, PsyD, PhD, serves as a psychotherapist for adolescents and adults in conjunction with his role as an academic researcher. He published over 100 articles on clinical psychology, psychoanalysis, and psychiatry in international journals.

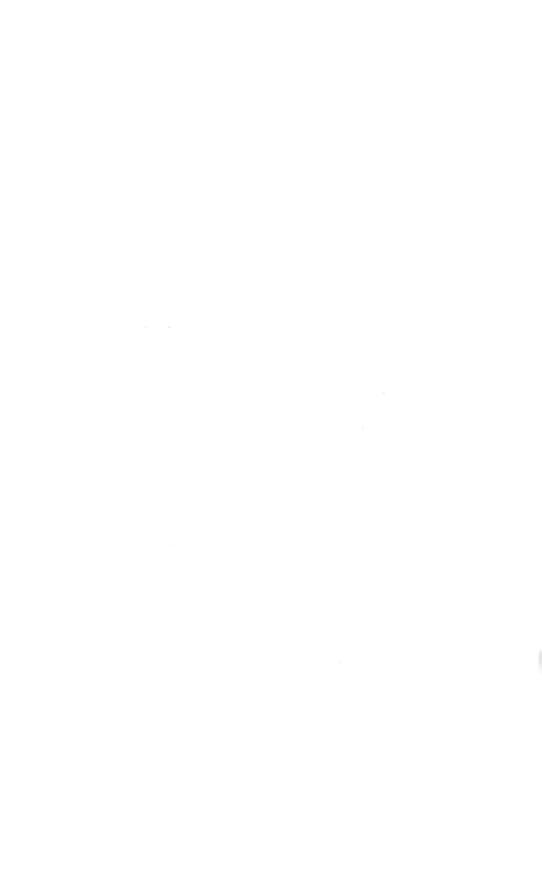

Contents

Figures

Foreword to Surrealism and Psychoanalysis in Grace Pailthorpe's life and work

Lee Ann Montanaro and Alberto Stefana

Grace Pailthorpe was an extraordinarily adventurous woman, qualifying as a doctor prior to World War I and serving in hospitals run by the Red Cross for the wounded from the trenches. Then after the war she pursued "adventures" in psychoanalysis, then criminology, and eventually surrealist painting. How much can one pack into a single life? Surviving a childhood being the only daughter with nine brothers seems, well, almost surreal in itself. It may well have instilled the idea that life was an adventure, both in the real world of war and medicine and in the internal world of the emotional unconscious and aesthetics.

This book is a professional biography and a companion to the previous publication, *Grace Pailthorpe's Writings on Psychoanalysis and Surrealism*. That first volume by the same authors detailed much of Pailthorpe's painting and her self-analytic reflections on their unconscious meanings. And the present book can only make us wonder at the explorations Pailthorpe made, and the ground that can be covered in a single life. Also we can notice how the move towards exploring one's inner world gradually drew her away from a more public life with others. That solitariness has led to the relative neglect of her work in the fields that she explored.

In spite of her withdrawal, Pailthorpe was actually an accomplished activist in all her areas of interest. These ranged from her medical work to the organisations she created within the early development of criminology where she campaigned to replace "purposeless punishment" with "compassionate justice," and then to the considerable output of writing within psychoanalysis, and eventually to the equally considerable aesthetic output of paintings from age 50 until she died, aged 87.

Interestingly, despite her withdrawal, Pailthorpe's psychoanalytic studies of the mental states of patients and of herself, retained a public activism. She created organisations in criminology, as well as lecturing on how to expose internal mental states as physical presences in the form of paintings. Her art remains of significant value at the auction houses today. Inspired and partnered by Reuben Mednikoff, from 1935, she used surrealist painting to give an enduring *physical* existence to *inner* impulses and experiences. This activity giving external manifestations of inner states is called "automatism," a word used in the late-nineteenth century and early twentieth century initially within spiritualism. But it spread to other domains of interest and was eventually adopted by the French surrealists.

Andre Breton, around whom Surrealism had developed, used automatic *writing* as a creative method for literature. Clearly, Pailthorpe and Mednikoff were in the same "automatist" vein, although they were not perhaps the first to give art a psychological purpose. Indeed, we can read that Jung is to be included in a long tradition that encouraged mental health patients to express their internal world in this automatist way. At the time, the acquaintance with Klein's ideas on the earliest phases of a baby's development influenced Pailthorpe's "play" with art materials. Children too use drawing actively and almost compulsively to give expression to their earliest creativity. Their play with toys is also a parallel automatism, using toys to play out their unconscious phantasies in the form of "automatic" drama, a theatrical automatism. These various methods of accessing hidden aspects of the mind supplement Freud's initial method based on free association with the elements of dreams. Similarly, in recent adult psychoanalysis, there is an increasing focus on the roles played out by analyst and analysand in the dramas of the primitive transference-countertransference relationships.

Pailthorpe's intentions bridged two worlds, that of art where she is valued, and that of psychoanalysis where she is largely forgotten (although we read that Marion Milner had once been intrigued by Pailthorpe's work). That bridge between creative art and psychoanalysis was explored in theoretical terms by Herbert Read, Roger Fry, Clive Bell, and others, but Pailthorpe achieved a *practical* method of exploration. Despite that, her contribution to the bridge has been rarely followed up. This does not mean that her bridging work is not valuable in solving the mystery of human creativity. This book does a service in calling attention again to Pailthorpe's activist approach to a problem yet to be solved.

Pailthorpe's enthusiastic use of a psychoanalytic model to squeeze conclusions from her paintings was based on Otto Rank's pre-Oedipal notion of "birth trauma." Giving such importance to the separation that birth itself implies rendered Rank one of the early analysts deviating from Freud's Oedipus complex. His non-conformism might well have appealed to Pailthorpe brought up in the extreme gospel hall tradition of the non-conforming Plymouth Brethren church. Moreover, Rank during a period living in Paris became the analyst of some of the creative circle there in the 1930s, including Henry Miller and Anais Nin.

The psychoanalytic principles and ideas relevant to Pailthorpe's practice were influenced by her context, the British psychoanalytic school and in particular its dominant figure in the 1930s, Melanie Klein. Like Klein, (and Klein's first analyst Sàndor Ferenczi) she regarded the new-born infant as having an ego (that is, a personality) from the very beginning, at birth, although of a very primitive kind. This diverged from Freud who considered there was a developmental phase before the infant found itself having a "self." For Freud, in that phase, the baby does not differentiate itself from the outside world. It is a state he called "narcissism." Interestingly, Pailthorpe anticipated Winnicott's later terminology when she debated the infant's struggle to distinguish the "me" from the "not-me" experiences. Indeed, Winnicott may also have been influenced in developing the squiggle game with children, a game which resembles Pailthorpe's methodology closely.

That debate over the exact timing when the personality emerges remains unresolved today, and Pailthorpe's claim for her work as scientific evidence would not necessarily be endorsed. Nevertheless, the very early ego stressed by Rank and Pailthorpe is echoed much more recently by the Italian child psychotherapist, Alessandra Piontelli, who published (in 1992) *intra-uterine* observations of 11 foetuses.

What Grace Pailthorpe has left us with is rather tantalising. The book is almost entirely a professional biography and it hardly touches on her personal life and relationships. I guess that has been deliberate by the authors, but also, I reckon Pailthorpe was very private and left few traces of the intimate details of her life. One wonders about her close relationship with Mednikoff. Were they purely painting partners? That cannot be, I think. When he changed his name to Richard Pailthorpe that is a declaration of… something. Intriguingly, it is the name of her great-nephew. And Pailthorpe and Mednikoff then presented themselves as brother and sister, even though the age difference between them was 23 years. It fills one's head with question marks. Why change his name; and why in 1948? All this is probably not known. Or is there a third book for someone to write, still buried in the archives? It is curious that Pailthorpe is emphatic that the earliest thoughts, feelings, and reactions determine adult life. But having exposed in her painting her earliest experiences, she then seems so closed about the consequent adult life she had.

The present book has been an exhaustive work to rescue what can be known more than fifty years since Grace Pailthorpe died in 1971. She was an extraordinary person, devoted to an extraordinary mission. She was tirelessly intent on exposing the earliest of our experiences as both psychologically powerful and also at the very root of human creativity.

Bob Hinshelwood – June 2023

Piontelli, A. (1992). *From Foetus to Child: An Observational and Psychoanalytic Study*. London: Routledge.

Acknowledgements

This biography pieces together the life of Grace Pailthorpe so sincere appreciation goes to the families of Grace Pailthorpe and Reuben Mednikoff. These family members include Grace Pailthorpe's nephew, David Bruce Pailthorpe, and great nephew, Richard Pailthorpe, for providing the insightful conversations about Pailthorpe's family. Gratitude must also be given to Reuben Mednikoff's nephew, Tony Black, for his insight into the professional and private lives of the couple.

Extreme appreciation is also granted to Professor Emeritus Robert Hinshelwood from the University of Essex who played an essential role in this project due to his consistent professional support, enthusiasm, and personal interest in the life and work of Grace Pailthorpe. Professor Emeritus Elizabeth Cowling's (University of Edinburgh) supervision of the research on the life of Grace Pailthorpe is sincerely appreciated together with the Edinburgh Dean Gallery archivist Kirstie Meehan who provided immediate access to the archive's contents.

Glenn Gossling from the Tavistock and Portman NHS Foundation Trust also shared his expertise on Grace Pailthorpe's close connection to the Portman Clinic. A final thank you in the compilation of the images is due to the art collector Viktor Wynd from the Last Tuesday Society and to the photographer Luke Walker.

Introduction

This book is intended both for lay readers of psychoanalytic or art history, as well as students and experts in these fields. As far as possible when discussing psychoanalytic theories, we have tried to outline concepts and ideas in modern day language. The book describes Grace Pailthorpe's life and original contribution to art and psychoanalysis. She was an English surgeon, specialist in psychological medicine, criminologist, associate member of the British PsychoAnalytical Society, and an artist. Although today Pailthorpe is recognised by art historians as a significant British surrealist painter of the twentieth century (Maclagan, 1998; Remy, 1999; Rosemont, 1998; Walsh & Wilson, 1998; Wolf, 2019), she was initially a relatively obscure figure whose work was barely recognised by her peers and scarcely acknowledged by historians of psychoanalysis.

Pailthorpe was born on 29 July 1883. She had a strict puritanical, Christian upbringing which she eventually rebelled against. Pailthorpe began her studies in medicine in 1908 and received her Bachelor of Medicine and Surgery (University of Durham) in 1914 at the age of 31.

Pailthorpe served in the French and British Red Cross during World War I. Her work with war victims encouraged her to study psychoanalysis and she started her training with Ernest Jones in 1923. That same year Pailthorpe also began her study on female offenders with the criminologist Maurice Hamblin Smith. This study led to the formation of the Institute of the Scientific Treatment of Delinquency in 1931 and the publication of *Studies in the Psychology of Delinquency* and *What We Put in Prison* in 1932. She also extended her research on delinquency in Kenya and South Africa in 1934.

Early in 1935, Pailthorpe met the artist Reuben Mednikoff and they then began a collaborative project based on her psychoanalytic interpretation of their surrealist-like art works. Within the next few years, she developed the theory of birth trauma and presented their research in an article published in the *London Bulletin* entitled "The Scientific Aspect of Surrealism" (1938–39). Their art was exhibited in several galleries all over the world and people called it, "the best and most truly Surrealist" by André Breton at the International Surrealist exhibition of 1936 (Walsh & Wilson, 1998). However, partly because of the couple's refusal to only exhibit and publish with the support of the

DOI: 10.4324/9781003427032-1

British Surrealist group, they left for America in 1940 and never associated themselves with any other group.

Pailthorpe founded the Association for the Scientific Treatment of Delinquency in 1943 while in British Colombia. Its focus was also juvenile delinquency. The attention gained because of the Association's approach to art therapy led to the birth of Canadian Surrealism. Pailthorpe and Mednikoff returned to England in 1946 where she then devoted the rest of her life to her work as an artist and analyst. Her last exhibition was held in Hastings in 1969 and she died two years later.

Much of our research and facts are based on conversations with family members of both Pailthorpe and Mednikoff together with archival material that is found at Modern Two (formerly the Dean Gallery) archive in Edinburgh. There is also less material on Pailthorpe's work after her return to London with Mednikoff in 1946 since they withdrew from public life. One significant factor to take into consideration when reading this biography is that Pailthorpe was a very private person and there is very little information on her personal relationships. She remained committed to her research throughout her life.

The book adopts a chronological and narrative historical approach to Pailthorpe's life and career. It outlines six main phases: from her birth until the period just after the end of her service as a surgeon during the Great War (1883–1922; Chapter 1); from the start of both her psychoanalytic training and the study of female offenders until the end of her ethnocultural-oriented research in Africa (1923–34; Chapters 3 and 4); from the first meeting with Reuben Mednikoff until the end of their association with the British surrealist movement (1935–40; Chapters 7, 8, 9, and 10); the period the couple spent in North America (1941–46; Chapter 11); the couple's return to London (1946–mid-1950s; Chapter 12); and the remainder of Pailthorpe's life (Chapter 13). Chapter 2 gives an insight into Mednikoff's life before he met Pailthorpe in 1935. Chapters 5 and 6 outline the relationship between psychoanalysis and Surrealism.

1   Early life

Grace Winifred Pailthorpe was born in St. Leonard's-on-Sea in Sussex on 29 July 1883. She was the third child and only girl as she had nine brothers. Her father, Edward Pailthorpe, was a prominent stockbroker and her mother, Anne Lavinia nee Green, was a seamstress. Because of the Plymouth Brethren practices, Pailthorpe and her brothers were educated at their home in Redhill, Surrey by tutors. This was because home-schooling would prevent them from being indoctrinated by the outside world Richard Pailthorpe,[1] personal communication with Lee Ann Montanaro, 2008. As she recalled, "we liked to play instead of pray, we liked to make a noise when we should engage in silent worship, we liked all the things of this world, when it is expressly forbidden so to do" (Pailthorpe, 1925). Though, when older, Pailthorpe often spoke about the nightmares her childhood gave her, postcards written by her father just before his death in 1904 indicate the strong bond between them. After his death, Pailthorpe's family moved to Southport in Lancashire. They also spent their holidays in Scotland in a rented house (the identity of the owners is unknown) called St. Germains on the road to North Berwick and Musselburgh.

Just like her relationship with her father, Pailthorpe was also very close to her younger brother Alexander, who was known as Frank. They were close in age and thinking. Neither of them had a good relationship with their mother, who by all accounts was very dictatorial and this was probably because, as children, they must have questioned their Plymouth Brethren upbringing which was "incomprehensibly destructive" (Richard Pailthorpe, personal communication with Lee Ann Montanaro, 2008). Unlike Frank (who was killed in action in 1915 during World War I) and her, Pailthorpe's other siblings were only married into the Brethren. All of her brothers' children were also brought up as Plymouth Brethren and remained tied to it for some time.

It is likely that Pailthorpe became interested in pursuing a medical career partly because her paternal aunt Mary Elizabeth was a doctor and had achieved much by qualifying in the 1880s when there were very few female doctors. Mary was a medical missionary, so in her case religion came into the equation whereas Pailthorpe herself never seemed to have considered working

DOI: 10.4324/9781003427032-2

as a missionary. Due to her aunt's profession, it is unlikely that there would have been much opposition to Pailthorpe also having a career in medicine.

Pailthorpe attended the London (Royal Free Hospital) School of Medicine for Women in the Winter term of 1908–09. She qualified as Bachelor of Medicine and Bachelor of Surgery (MBBS) at the University of Durham in 1914 at the age of 31. Of the 34 graduates of MBBS in the calendar year 1914, Pailthorpe was one of three females. Of 66 graduates in all medical degrees (MD, MS, MBBS, DPH, LDS) that year, she was one of only four females. These statistics show how rare it was for a woman to study medicine at the time.

Shortly after the outbreak of war on 28 July 1914, Pailthorpe rushed to London because she wanted to volunteer her service (4 August 1914). However, after submitting her application form at the War Office, officials told her that they did not favour the inclusion of female medics and rejected her offer. Still, after completing her degree in medicine and surgery where she was awarded an honours, Pailthorpe registered on 21 December 1914 and went on to serve in the French and British Red Cross during World War I. Despite the fact that applications by female medics were initially routinely rejected, "Before 2 years had elapsed there were over a thousand women medicals on active service on every front" (A62/1/025).

Although many medical records were destroyed in the 1940 air raids, records relating to Pailthorpe's military service in the British army during the war can be traced and, because of this, we know that she served as a surgeon in several different hospitals between 1915 and 1918. In January 1915, at the start of her military service, she worked as a surgeon with the Bromley-Martin Hospital Unit in the Haute-Marne District in France. As she described in her journal, the staff she worked with had all been rejected by the military authorities in their applications because of their sex, age, or health. The staff, among others, consisted of three artists, a sculptor, a poet, an architect, and a historian. Pailthorpe was in charge of several wards and acted as a personal assistant to the chief medical officer, Dr. Aspland, who had worked as a gynecologist and missionary in Peking before the war.

Between August and October 1916, Pailthorpe worked as a surgeon in Salonika in the Royal Army Medical Corps of the British Committee of the French Red Cross. Several photos of this period show us that Pailthorpe then spent some time in Malta and there is also evidence that on 12 December 1916, Pailthorpe was granted leave by the Governor of Malta to proceed to Italy. She boarded the S. S. "Isonzo for Adriatic" on 13 December. A year later, while she was based in France, Pailthorpe set up the "Amiens Club" for the soldiers. It first came into being in Amiens in October 1917 and was named "Home from Home." Half of the staff Pailthorpe worked with were artists themselves, so they must have influenced her early interest in art. Sometime later, she was transferred from the French to the British Red Cross and worked as a District Medical Officer at Queen Charlotte's Hospital in London. She remained in London until the end of the war and worked as a

House Physician at Charing Cross Hospital, an Assistant Medical Officer at Whipps Cross War Hospital and finally, as a House Physician at London Hospital. As her war journal clarifies, it was Pailthorpe's experience as a doctor for victims of the war that led her to a lifetime practice of psychological medicine (Montanaro, 2010).

Pailthorpe's poor relationship with her mother is further emphasised in her autobiographical notes as she wrote how her mother, who died towards the end of the war in 1918, had not left Pailthorpe a share of the inheritance money in her will and instead left everything to her sons. Pailthorpe was considering changing faith to Catholicism and this would, no doubt, have upset her mother because of her strict Plymouth Brethren beliefs. Pailthorpe's autobiographical notes confirm how bitter her mother's will made her feel since it resulted in her having little money to finance her career. Ironically, most of her brothers squandered their inheritance (Richard Pailthorpe, personal communication with Lee Ann Montanaro, 2009).

Once the war ended, Pailthorpe decided to visit her brother, Douglas, in Australia (she left for her destination on 11 December 1918) with her friend, Mary Aeldrin Cullis who, like her, was "addicted to travelling" (Pailthorpe, 1920–22). The manuscript of her unpublished travel journal, entitled *Truants* shows that their plan to go to Australia came about because they believed that, after the war, a holiday and a change of scenery were necessary. *Truants* is dated 1920 to 1922, and like her autobiographical notes, it is partly written in the form of reminiscences. The two friends left for their destination on 11 December 1918 and arrived in Fremantle on 10 February 1919.

Pailthorpe's purpose in travelling to Australia seems to have been a combination of visiting her brother, sightseeing and developing her career, which for a female doctor at that time may not have been so easy in Britain. It is likely that it was during this period that she first became interested in criminology as, historically, criminals had often been shipped to Australia because their transportation was seen as a humane alternative to execution.

Between 1919 and 1921, Pailthorpe worked as a general physician and a district medical officer of a large area with headquarters in the Youanmi gold mine (Australia), where a moving train sometimes served as temporary surgery. Additionally, she earned travelling expenses by working as a general physician in New Zealand. At the time, there was very little encouragement for women to build professional careers for themselves so it would have been very unusual for a foreign woman to become a Medical Officer of Health. Because of this, any female doing medicine at that time needed to be both intelligent and strong enough to succeed in a largely male-dominated environment. Although as she wrote in *Truants*, Pailthorpe was liked by the patients, she felt the pressure from her local colleagues and was not popular with the midwives as she considered them to be indifferent or cynical about their work (Pailthorpe, 1920–22).

Following her practice in Australia and New Zealand, Pailthorpe and Cullis travelled to Hawaii, Vancouver, and New York between 20 October 1921 and 7 February 1922. They then returned to Southampton.

Note

1 Richard Pailthorpe is Grace Pailthorpe's great nephew. His grandfather was her brother.

2   Reuben Mednikoff

Since Reuben Mednikoff (1906–1934) played a major role in Pailthorpe's life, it is important to provide an account of the life, intellectual and artistic development, and career of Mednikoff before meeting her in 1935. Therefore, this chapter outlines his childhood, education, love experiences, early career as a designer of advertisements and as a poet, and his discovery of Surrealism and psychoanalysis. Unlike Pailthorpe, who had many years of professional life and already had a public profile by the time they met in 1935, Mednikoff's early life is shrouded in obscurity. Professionally, there is almost no information about his early work, hardly any illustrations of it, and an almost complete lack of critical reviews of these works. This absence of evidence means that there are long stretches of his life about which next to nothing is known. More so, it is difficult to define a stylistic evolution of his art before he met Pailthorpe in 1935 since there are only a few sources that shed light on Mednikoff's early art career apart from his highly subjective memoirs.

Mednikoff was born on 2 June 1906 at his parents' house at 4, Morgan Houses, Hessel Street, Tower Hamlets, London. His father, Myer, a tinplate worker, and his mother, Annie née Walter, registered his birth on 16 July 1906 in the Eastern 54 sub-district of St George and St John in London. He was the fourth child of a Jewish family of Russian immigrant origin and his relationship with his family and his childhood experiences were crucial to the development of his artistic career as they always remained vivid to him. Many people from Eastern Europe moved to the West at the end of the nineteenth century for a variety of reasons, but mostly due to religious persecution. Many Jews settled in the East End of London around the inner-city working-class districts of Whitechapel and Stepney, close to where their ships had docked. Conversations with Mednikoff's nephew, Tony Black, reveal that although Mednikoff's parents were born in Russia, they moved to Whitechapel towards the end of the nineteenth century probably because of the large-scale wave of anti-Jewish pogroms.

The impact of the notorious May Laws of 1882 under the reign of Alexander III led to restrictions on Jewish land ownership, the prohibition of trading on Christian holidays, and the prevention of Jews from settling in

DOI: 10.4324/9781003427032-3

villages or studying in secular schools. Despite there being no information as to which part of Russia Mednikoff's family originated from, Mednikoff and his three sisters and two brothers were all born in London in an area which was notorious for much poverty, homelessness, prostitution, exploitive work conditions and infant mortality. Initially, his grandparents also came to Britain but decided to return to Russia.

The early years of Mednikoff seem to have been very troubled. A fall at the age of two resulted in Mednikoff suffering from unusually severe headaches throughout his life, and because he discussed this fall with his sister Milly in letters they sent to one another from December 1935 to February 1936, it is certain that he became deeply engrossed in psychoanalysis in the mid-30s. This was probably because he believed that psychoanalysis would enable him to confront his personal problems better and give meaning to his private anxieties. Furthermore, several of Mednikoff's paintings reveal that many of his motifs sprang from his Jewish childhood experiences. The densely populated and poor conditions of Jewish neighbourhoods in London meant that these quarters developed into the perfect breeding grounds for fascism and communism and became Britain's most politicised areas.

Despite this, the safety that Britain offered from persecution was a better alternative than staying in the Jew-hating societies of Eastern Europe. In his essay "The unconscious is always right," Andrew Wilson described how, as a child, Mednikoff rebelled against any form of orthodox religion and was beaten by the local rabbi because he hated praying as "it was a continual reminder of killing." His revulsion is revealed in his work *Come Back Soon* (1936) as it details the horror of Jewish slaughterhouses. Mednikoff's rebellion also brings Pailthorpe's rebellion against the Plymouth Brethren religion to mind, even though she did not experience violence.

At the age of seven, Mednikoff began his education at Eleanor Road School in London and reached Standard VII. He was described as being well-behaved, intelligent, industrious, reliable, honest, and punctual by the school's headmaster T. G. Dixon. However, his early enthusiasm for painting received little encouragement. He asked for permission to study art when he was only 13, but his parents told him that studying business would be wiser. During this time, for the majority of British-born working-class Jews, financial constraints meant that there were few opportunities to remain in education beyond the age of 14, and so they would leave school with only an elementary education. Boys would then be expected to enter full-time employment.

Despite the initial opposition of his parents, Mednikoff was enrolled at St Martin's School of Art in 1920 at the age of 14. It is possible that since his family was not wealthy, he had obtained a scholarship, but there is no record of any such award. Founded in 1854, St Martin's School of Art was firmly established as one of the leading fine art and commercial art schools in England. Boys from the age of 13 onwards were admitted, and classes involved drawing, painting and modelling from life, poster designing, geometrical drawing, outdoor sketching, and landscape composition. Unfortunately, none of his work as a student has come to light. The academic calendar of St Martin's School of Art shows that Mednikoff studied there until 1923. It is difficult to trace the development of Mednikoff's work from 1923 till his meeting with Pailthorpe, as so little of it is known, but press cuttings, letters, and exhibition catalogues show that he painted and wrote poetry throughout these years.

In addition to his medical history, Mednikoff's experience of love may also have prompted his interest in psychoanalysis. Although no records relating to his early sexual development have surfaced, a marriage certificate proves that Mednikoff married Marie Louise de Sousa on 14 December 1932, at the Register Office in Hampstead. However, nothing is known about de Sousa's social or national background. Though arranged marriages were customary among Jewish families at the time, there is no information on how or where the couple met. Following their marriage, they moved to 28, Belsize Square, Hampstead. Soon after, de Sousa had an affair with Mednikoff's friend Harold Botcherby. After admitting it to him, De Sousa left Mednikoff as she was pregnant. Their marriage was dissolved on 28 January 1935.

Though there is no evidence that Mednikoff experienced psychoanalysis prior to meeting Pailthorpe, his knowledge of Surrealism through his connection with the poet David Gascoyne in 1933 makes it evident that he was aware of the influence of Freudian psychoanalysis on Surrealism by that time. Most likely, one of the major influences on Mednikoff's early artistic and intellectual career was Hampstead itself. Hampstead was a substantially developed area and had established its reputation as a healthy and attractive place to stay because of its fresher air, pleasant views, and its sense of separation from central London. Britain in the 1930s was in economic and social turmoil because of the slump and the threat of war. Aesthetic discussions were engulfed in new theories and movements, with artists being caught up in political and social uncertainties. They turned Hampstead into the headquarters for avant-garde art of every stamp. It was "the cradle of the modern movement in English art," and its residents included left-wing intellectuals, writers, and a group of committed modernist artists such as Roland Penrose, Ben Nicholson, Henry Moore, Herbert Read, Barbara Hepworth, and Christopher Nevinson.

Furthermore, the Nazi persecution of the Jews sent many artists into exile and several émigrés moved to Britain because they were fleeing religious persecution and totalitarian regimes. Walter Gropius, Eric Mendelshon, Marcel Breuer, Naum Gabo, and Maholy-Nagy all took up residence in Hampstead in the 1930s. Other famous artists of Jewish descent living in London were Mark Gertler, Jacob Epstein, and William Rothenstein. Their parents, like Minkoff's, were all Jewish immigrants. These artists belonged to an earlier generation and there is no firm evidence that Mednikoff had had any personal contact with them, but it is likely that he benefited from their example and was following a route that had already been mapped out. For example, Epstein's controversial topics were characterised by the themes of maternity, commemoration, and religious suffering and were inspired by the Jewish community in East London. Similar themes are seen in Mednikoff's work. Epstein's works display an expressive distortion of the human figure, and this is often seen in Mednikoff's drawings and paintings in the 1930s. Epstein's sculpture *Woman Possessed* (1932), for instance, can be compared to the three-dimensional form in Mednikoff's *The Stairway to Paradise* (1936).

A significant friend and influence for Mednikoff in the early 1930s was David Gascoyne. A letter, dated 23 March 1933, confirms that Mednikoff's friend, Elizabeth Tregaskis, asked Mednikoff to visit her as Gascoyne was anxious to meet him. This shows that Gascoyne was well acquainted with Mednikoff's writings and drawings. In fact, Gascoyne even gave a copy of his poem, *Slate*, to Mednikoff.

Soon after meeting Gascoyne, Mednikoff exhibited four drawings, four landscape watercolours and another two watercolours entitled *Cactus* and *Conscious to the Subconscious* at the exhibition "Today's Art" at the Keane Galleries in London in May 1933. He signed these works "Reuben." The paintings were for sale and five were sold. The exhibition catalogue shows that two of the watercolours were bought by Sidney Schiff Esq. whereas *Cactus*, *Conscious to the Subconscious*, and another watercolour were bought by Mrs. Hayter Preston. There is no information on Sidney Schiff, but Hayter Preston was the wife of the literary editor of the *Sunday Referee*. Today, all of these works' whereabouts are unknown but, at the time, particularly *Cactus* and *Conscious to the Subconscious*, received praise in the *Sunday Referee*. The newspaper also illustrated an image of *Cactus* and, when referring to it, an anonymous reviewer wrote:

> One of the finest paintings in the exhibition is a large decoration – Cactus – by an artist who disguises himself under the name of Reuben. I cannot understand why an artist should follow the fashion of caricaturists, jazz drummers, and dictators, in using one name only. Reuben is a painter of great originality, with a bold imagination, an artistic daring, and a fine paint quality at his disposal. His "Cactus" decoration is one of the most interesting works I have seen for a long time.

The art critic also described *Conscious to the Subconscious* as a "non-representational design that is best to allocate the title to the category of unsolved mysteries, and to be content with appraising the suggestive form and colour of a work which is boldly realised and firmly handled." The title *Conscious to the Subconscious* points towards the influence of Surrealism on Mednikoff and their shared interest in the psychoanalytic theories of Freud.

Poems by both Gascoyne and Mednikoff were published in the poetry section, "The Poet's Corner," of the *Sunday Referee* between 1933 and 1934. Victor Neuberg edited this weekly column. Tharp, who was also known by her maiden name Sheila Macleod, was the column's sub-editor. "The Poet's Corner" first appeared in April 1933 but was brought to an end due to the reorganisation of the *Sunday Referee* in November 1935.

The two of Mednikoff's poems which were published in "The Poet's Corner" are:

Acquiescence Tradition

The saturated aspect of a wide City
street
The grey-sad silhouette of a tree,
lopped of all branches,
against a background of rising stone.
The abject submission is felt in the
very angle at which the trunk
falls
to meet the earth ...
but stamps of all that had been
branches
still persist
in raising their cropped heads
to the sky.
Tradition, maternal spirit, is an harlot unsuspected ...
feathering away the dust of cosmic years from memories cold storaged in
time..
coaxing with procurant eyes aged souls to untimely seeding ...
with senile eyes watching frail thought unseemly straining in forgotten
dust.
This vigourless moiety, from wearied age reborn, is uncomely
and too soon do time's disintegrating fingers tatter the vital strain.
Can limbs without life still mock the gestures of agonised pain
or vision the warmth they would kindle in frigid veins?
Or does Death, the toothless scoundrel, desire
a more brittle bone to ease his labouring gums?

Acquiescence was published on 1 October 1933 and *Tradition* was published on 2 December 1934. The quality of the imagery, content, and structure of *Acquiescence* and *Tradition* proves that Mednikoff was already influenced by Surrealism. Both poems convey a lyrical element of human thought, and his use of free verse allows the structure to follow a looser pattern than what would be expected in a traditional form. It is an open-ended poetry freed from the normal confines of logical structure as it portrays an irrational stream-of-consciousness.

In *Acquiescence*, Mednikoff abandons himself to the meandering flow of thought as he views the landscape whereas, in *Tradition* he breaks clauses into fragments. In both poems, Mednikoff manipulates words and images, turning them into subjects of reflection. Both poems contain the displacement that is associated with Surrealist poetry, and there is an interplay between conscious perception and dream. The extended metaphors in his poems appear to work through the accumulation of observed details, and this visual description derives in part from Mednikoff's recognition that images are an element common to both waking and sleeping states.

Mednikoff's use of automatic writing is evident in *Acquiescence*, as the text consists of two long sentences. The juxtaposition of verbal elements such as the earth and the wind as described in the poem permeate the lyrics. The events that appear before the questioning gaze of the subject hint at some displaced meaning. On the other hand, as Gascoyne's *Slate*, *Tradition* presents the reader with a morbid setting that depicts a painful isolation within a homeless environment. Like Gascoyne, Mednikoff writes in a form that eliminates end rhyme. The concreteness of the sensory detail is anchored within a grammar that reinforces the mystery of the monologue. The fusion of description, narration, and setting blurs the distinction between the conscious and the unconscious. As seen, the techniques of Mednikoff and Gascoyne evoke the enigmatic qualities of things by placing them in eerie surroundings or a verbally created scene. Their dominating visual details create settings that are oddly dream-like in that the visual imagery is grounded in a precise observation of natural detail, yet the uninterrupted accumulation of those details form settings that seem to emerge from a dream and encompass the external world.

"The Poet's Corner" was a resounding success and other poets whom Mednikoff befriended and who also published their works in the column included Dylan Thomas (who was the second recipient of the poetry prize), Julian Symons, Pamela Hansford Johnson, Edward Milne, Herbert Corby, Idris Davies, Leslie Daiken, Laurie Lee and Ruthven Campbell Todd. Moreover, Gascoyne's membership in the Surrealist movement and his association with its leading members placed him in an ideal position to witness and record the development of its leading writers and artists. Thus, it was probably through Gascoyne that Mednikoff became involved with the first stirrings of Surrealism in England, as letters in the Edinburgh archive (dated 1933 to 1936) show us that they often corresponded and had several friends in common.

On Monday 17 September 1934, Mednikoff started working for Norfolk Studio Ltd. This was a company of designers and copywriters of advertisements. A letter from Norfolk Studio to Mednikoff proves that the latter had prepared some illustrations and shown them to the director, who then offered him the job. Whilst working at Norfolk Studio, Mednikoff exhibited 20 drawings and paintings at another exhibition at the Keane Galleries in London. The exhibition opened on 23 November 1934. The exhibition catalogue states that Mednikoff's works were on sale and the prices ranged from £3 to £15. The fate of the majority is unknown, but they were praised in

The Times (29.11.34) by Charles Marriott, who claimed that "Besides having good taste in colour, well shown in the still-life painting of "Bowl and the small 'Landscape,' Mednikoff is an excellent draughtsman, realising his effects – including recession – with great economy of means. The studies of the dog 'Patch' and the landscapes 'Hedges' and 'Devon Lane' may be quoted." In contrast to his previous exhibition, this review and the titles of the works suggest that they were not markedly Surrealist in imagery or style. What is clear, however, is that Mednikoff's art was gaining positive critical attention.

Even before the famous 1936 International Surrealist exhibition, Surrealism had already caused some stir in magazines and newspapers in London. April 1933 saw the reopening of the Mayor Gallery marked by an exhibition of the works of Miró, Ernst, Klee, Picabia, and Arp, and another Ernst exhibition was mounted a year later. The Zwemmer Gallery featured Dalí's first two exhibitions in London in the Spring and Autumn of 1934. Given the familiarity with Surrealist imagery and the practice of automatism revealed in Mednikoff's poems, and his friendship with Gascoyne, it is highly likely that he saw these exhibitions and thus had firsthand knowledge of Surrealist theory, poetry, and art before he first met Pailthorpe in February 1935. Moreover, Mednikoff's work for Norfolk Studio lasted for no more than a few months, as he left his job soon after meeting Pailthorpe. By leaving so rapidly, he may have been influenced by his awareness of the deep disapproval of the Surrealists of all forms of commercial art.

In December 1935, Mednikoff wrote to Gascoyne proposing himself as a reviewer of *A short survey of Surrealism*. Gascoyne replied that, much as he would have liked this to happen, another reviewer had already been chosen. It is most likely that Mednikoff first heard about the 1936 International Surrealist exhibition from Gascoyne, as, in the same letter, Gascoyne wrote:

Did you know that there is to be a very large surrealist exhibition at the Burlington Galleries next June? I do hope you'll be up in town to see it. André Breton and Paul Eluard are to visit London and deliver various lectures. Salvador Dalí is to visit London at about the same time, and is having a show of his own at Lefevres (...) We hope to be able to bring out an occasional English surrealist "bulletin" during 1936. I'll let you know whether this comes out (...) It seems I haven't seen any of our mutual friends for a long time.

Therefore, it seems that Mednikoff's and Pailthorpe's invitation to participate in the International Surrealist exhibition in 1936 occurred through Gascoyne. Gascoyne's awareness of Mednikoff's research with Pailthorpe is illustrated in this letter as he ended it by saying: "What is it exactly that you are doing down there in Cornwall? Research work? It sounds most exciting and mysterious. Do write to me (...) and let me know more about yourself."

Another letter from Gascoyne to Mednikoff, written on 20 July 1936, also reveals their close relationship and their common interests:

> I imagine you both to be hard at work in your seclusion, and am most interested to know how it is all going (...) Taking you at your word, I am wondering whether it would be possible for you and Dr. Pailthorpe to take me as a paying-guest for a few weeks, if convenient just now. You were kind enough to offer me your hospitality and, feeling in need of a change of air and scene, it would be most pleasant to stay with people with whom I share so much interest in common, and in such a congenial part of the country.

Clearly, unlike Pailthorpe, who was the daughter of a stockbroker and had travelled extensively, Mednikoff was the son of a poor tinplate worker, had spent most of his time in London, and then entered the commercial art world for financial reasons. He was very different from Pailthorpe in social class, age, temperament, religious background, and professional training. However, his quick understanding of the use and interpretation of symbols in art motivated Pailthorpe to further research of the unconscious and made her see him as the most suitable colleague for the research. Furthermore, at the time of their meeting, his art and poetry were already attracting attention and receiving praise from critics and friends alike. Thus, in spite of their differences, each complemented the other in talent and knowledge, and, through a process of deliberate absorption, may be said to have completed each other, eventually forming an indissoluble unit.

3 The study of female offenders and training in psychoanalysis

Early on in her career, Pailthorpe served as a surgeon in several different hospitals in the French and British Red Cross during World War I. These experiences with victims of war and her work as a general practitioner encouraged her to study psychoanalysis following her travels and return to England in February 1922. Pailthorpe sought Ernest Jones, the then president of the British Psychoanalytical Society and editor of the *International Journal of Psychoanalysis*, because he was recognised as the first person to develop the therapeutic practice of psychoanalysis in Britain. She decided to undergo training analysis with him and started doing so in 1923 (until 1930), and in the same year she became an associate member of the British Society.

Letters from Jones to Pailthorpe, dated from 25 December 1925 to 15 November 1932, show us that Jones encouraged Pailthorpe's analytic work a lot. In one of his letters to Pailthorpe, which was written just after her psychoanalytic sessions, Jones wrote:

Dear Dr Pailthorpe,

I was deeply moved by today's event. But I judged it would be more considerate not to introduce an emotional role into a situation you were holding so well in hand, especially as it did not mean any real parting. I count on seeing you again before long and so keeping touch with developments and with your news. In the meantime, however, I do want to convey to you some expression of my personal feeling for you. You must know actually how deeply bound I am with your fight for freedom and happiness and how greatly I care about your success. Your courage has never really faltered in all the tenacious battle, and this week I admired it more than ever. I am convinced it will not fail you in this particularly difficult time. Remember that the harder these things are to win the more valuable and precious are they when won, so there can never really be any doubt about if the fight is worthwhile.

Ernest Jones

(A62/1/001, 20 June 1930)

DOI: 10.4324/9781003427032-4

I am not the first person in your life to believe whole-heartedly in you, nor shall I be the last.

With heartfelt good wishes
Yours always

This letter shows us the degree of intimacy between the pair. Jones believed in the value of her work and they regularly communicated over the years.

In 1923, Pailthorpe also began her study on female offenders, working with and under the direction of Maurice Hamblin Smith. He believed psychoanalysis—which he saw as a "new development of psychology" (Hamblin Smith, 1922)—was a way of assessing the personality of offenders and a technique for treating the mental conflicts which, he claimed, lay behind the criminal act (Soothill et al., 2002). Hamblin Smith is identified as Britain's first authorised teacher of "criminology" (Garland, 1988) and the first individual to use the title of "criminologist" (Soothill et al., 2002). In July of that same year, the two colleagues published a joint paper entitled "Mental Tests for Delinquents: and Mental Conflicts as a Cause of Delinquency" (Hamblin Smith & Pailthorpe, 1923) in *The Lancet*. Their paper consisted of the results obtained from several mental tests which were carried out by both male and female prisoners in Birmingham Prison. They grouped the 325 cases under the headings of "normal," "subnormal," and "mentally defective." The subnormal group consisted of, "persons considered to be defective in intelligence" (*ivi*, p. 112), while the mentally defective group, "present all the criteria of permanent mental defect from an early age, with need for care, supervision, and control for their own protection or the protection of others" (ibid.). Both authors concluded that mental conflict was the single cause of delinquency:

> The welfare of society is of supreme importance. Our point is that these cases require treatment, in the interests of society as well as in their own, and that this treatment must be on special lines. What is wanted is: (a) recognition of these conflict cases by means of full investigation before trial; (b) appreciation by the courts of the value and the necessity of the treatment of these cases of conflict; (c) provision of means of treating these cases by (1) proper institutions, (2) perhaps some form of indeterminate sentence. (*ivi*, p. 114)

The work of Pailthorpe and Hamblin Smith was the first to introduce psychological and psychoanalytic ideas to the British penal system (Cordess, 1992). It is most likely that there were no other female criminologists working in the same field as Pailthorpe in Britain at this time and this makes her a pioneer not only in the theory and treatment of delinquency but also as a woman who, at the time, was still relatively young (Montanaro, 2010).

A year later, Pailthorpe also began her study on one hundred inmates of various Homes for girls and young women aged between 16 and 30 at the request of the Central Council for Preventive and Rescue Work in London (see Pailthorpe, 1926–27). Her research method was to interview the female prisoners individually as well as those who had been sent to Rescue and Preventive homes. The women were aged between 16 and 30 (A621/078, 10 September 1932). Pailthorpe would spend up to ten hours in conversation with each inmate and make as many as six or seven visits per case (A62/1/078, 20 September 1932). Whilst interviewing them, she wrote that although "at the time, my work was not to treat but to investigate, it was evident that many of the girls found considerable relief and often hope, when they discovered I was interested in their problems as they felt them, and not as society felt them" (Pailthorpe, 1920–29). Pailthorpe was mainly concerned with cases where she detected "mental conflict":

> As far as possible, one aimed at an outline of the life-history of the individual and her reactions to life. Her reactions to the present circumstances, her emotional mobility, her moods, the way in which she disposed of the situation in which she found herself (...) her mannerisms (...) habit spasms, tremors, blushing, sweating; (...) and her moods were all noted. Her history of states of depression and excitement was specially observed.
>
> (Pailthorpe, 1920–29)

Pailthorpe's notes and conclusions about her research show how her attitude to behaviour, emotions, and somatic symptoms of individuals with "mental conflicts" was influenced by her knowledge of Freud's works. Because the Viennese master considered hysteria to be more common amongst women, it is likely that his view influenced her decision to work with women. Moreover, although it is not clear whether or not she believed gender played a fundamental role in criminality, as a woman herself, Pailthorpe may have been more interested and sympathetic to female offenders.

In 1929, in the context of her research on young delinquents, Pailthorpe published in the *International Journal of Psychoanalysis* a review of the book *Autolycus or the Future for Miscreant Youth* by Ronald Grey Gordon, a British medical doctor who, similarly to Pailthorpe, served for four years as a captain in the Royal Army Medical Corps in France and the Middle East during the Great War. In her review, Pailthorpe draws attention to the conception of crime as something that varies in different countries and at different periods. Then she mentions the question of the personality of the delinquent, which according to Gordon is characterised by a conflict between the ego and the environment. She seems to agree with the author believing that the inability to adjust to the social order, and the underlying instability can be eliminated only "by the slow process of eugenic education" (Gordon, 1928, p. 37). The fact that educational, medical, psychological, and sociological conditions can be factors, secondary or otherwise, which lead to crime is also stated.

Pailthorpe underlines Gordon's reliance on Adlerian theory, according to which the sense of inferiority from mental retardation or physical defect in a youth involves a compensatory will to power and holds that delinquent conduct is often a manifestation of this overcompensation. Psychoanalysis, as believed by both the author and the reviewer, may do much for such youth, but it is too early to be sure of its positive or negative effects. Pailthorpe also showed her disagreement with Gordon on the importance given to the reconditioning of the external world as she believed the author was too optimistic in thinking that lasting psychological changes in the offender can be achieved just through such reconditioning.

With reference to Pailthorpe's own research, one can state that her contribution was original because she focused on the causes and prevention of criminality rather than on the punishment of the criminal. Pailthorpe was adamant that society must attempt to understand the unconscious motives at work behind all crime as she believed that offenders can only understand their offences if the unconscious motives prompting their behaviour have been made apparent to them. Pailthorpe wanted to implement psychoanalysis as a treatment and asserted that the prison conditions at that time were unsuitable for the reform of criminals.

Pailthorpe's (1932a) report for the Medical Research Council (MRC), titled *Studies in the Psychology of Delinquency*, maintains that in each case investigated there is an underlying pathological state of mind that should be treated through psychotherapeutic and re-educational interventions. She wanted to implement psychoanalysis as a treatment and asserted that the prison conditions at that time were unsuitable for the reform of criminals. The report sought to prove the great extent to which mental deficiency and instability are to blame for criminality. Pailthorpe focused on the cruelty and insufficiency of the penal system and presented new proposals on what action one can take, highlighting the importance of a psychological approach to the study of delinquency and its causes. However, as Edward Glover (1933) confirmed, this work was hampered by Pailthorpe's terms of reference and in several of its parts by the conditions under which the research was carried out as well as being subjected to much appraisal before publication (Montanaro, 2010).

Pailthorpe's (1932b) *What We Put in Prison* exceeds the above-mentioned limitations. This book drew on the findings of the MRC's report. It included descriptions of case histories as well as clinical-theoretical considerations which Pailthorpe recommended from a psychoanalytic perspective. Furthermore, her theories on delinquency now took on a more general slant and addressed criminality irrespective of gender. In the Author's note, Pailthorpe wrote: "if I can claim to be original at all in what I have presented, it is, perhaps, in focusing attention on the *law-makers* as having to come under investigation *in addition* to the law-breakers" (p. 1). In her book she maintained the idea of preventing crime by means of psychoanalysis. The offender's lifestyle would be examined and the offender would then be made to follow the typical lines of treatment by an analyst. Pailthorpe declared that psychoanalysis was the only cure for all psychological maladjustments: "It has been proved, again and again, that with psychoanalysis not only has the personality of an individual changed for the better, but also by the freeing of inhibitions and psychological difficulties, hitherto undiscovered, potential capacities have been released" (p. 153).

Pailthorpe professed that it was equally imperative to undertake research as a way of determining how beneficial the various methods of treatment were. She proposed the need for small laboratories where investigators would represent different schools of psychoanalysis so that tests would cover all the known methods of scientific treatment at the time. She identified the schools as those of Freud, Jung, and Adler. The investigator would select his cases and would be given the liberty to treat them since the respective individuals would fall under the guardianship of their investigator. She asserted that through this method, it would then be possible to establish the relative value of the various methods employed by each individual school of psychoanalysis by comparing the results the schools obtained for their respective cases (Pailthorpe, 1932b).

On 22 July 1931, a year before the publication of *Studies in the Psychology of Delinquency* and *What We Put in Prison*, Pailthorpe, Ernest Jensen, Victor Neuburg, and Runia Tharp formed the Association for the Scientific Treatment of Criminals (ASTC). Pailthorpe's report and book, which had been ready for publication since 1929, had provided the backing for the endeavours of the Committee and it was both Glover's and her initiative which had led to its establishment. The ASTC was renamed the Institute for the Scientific Treatment of Delinquency (ISTD) the following year. It was the first research Institute established in Britain that was dedicated to scientific research and treatment in the field of criminology (Jones, 2016).

The ISTD Committee set up a campaign to put Pailthorpe's recommendations into action. These were based on the terms of her report for the MRC (Pailthorpe, 1932a). The Committee decided to establish a body that would intensively study the psychology of, as well as offer psychotherapeutic treatment to, delinquents. As part of the treatment process of the ISTD, some of the patients made drawings and paintings which Pailthorpe believed expressed in symbolic form the desires of their unconscious. She analysed their drawings and used art as an instrument for psychological exploration, thus seeking an interactive relationship with her patients through painting. She related the forms and subjects of their art to their mental peculiarities as their compositions often portrayed incidents and conflicts in their lives. Here, Pailthorpe was using art as a diagnostic/therapeutic tool and her later encounter with the artist Reuben Mednikoff evidently motivated her into further research in this field.

In keeping up with the ISTD's aims (see Saville and Rumney, 1992) and with Pailthorpe's recommendation to set up small laboratories and establish

Remand Homes or Observation Centres, in 1933 the Institute opened the "Psychopathic Clinic," where Pailthorpe along with a group of psycho-analysts began treating delinquent and criminal patients through psycho-analytic psychotherapy. The first recorded appointment at the new clinical wing took place on 18 September 1933. The patient was a 47-year-old woman who was charged with assault on her female employer and required to receive help so she could control her violent temper (Portman Clinic, 2008). The "Psychopathic Clinic" was renamed the "Portman Clinic" in 1937 and it formally split from the ISTD and became part of the National Health Service in 1948 (Ruszczynski, 2016; Sarner, 2022).

Apart from Pailthorpe, the Institute's vice-presidents included Alfred Adler, Cyril Burt, Havelock Ellis, Sigmund Freud, the Lord Archbishop of York, Julian Huxley, The Very Rev. Hewlett Johnson (Dean of Canterbury), Ernest Jones, Carl Jung, Otto Rank, Viscount Templewood, the Countess De La Warr and H G Wells. Over the years, the group enlisted the support of some of the best-known psychologists in the world along with many British psychologists and psychotherapists. Together, they practised what they called "forensic psychotherapy"—a detailed, long-term treatment designed to help those who had nowhere else to go but back to prison—and they treated cases of habitual criminality, desperate addiction, extreme violence, and sexual perversion. All along, Pailthorpe insisted that no matter what measures were taken when examining delinquents or criminals, they must be balanced by intensive research and treatment with an intention to cure.

The resumé of Pailthorpe's book and report, issued by the ISTD in 1933, stated that Pailthorpe's "investigation demonstrates how, when these unfortunate people were approached from a scientific basis, eager-ness to co-operate in the understanding of their own problems was aroused" (Pailthorpe, 1928–34). It explained that Pailthorpe did not just discuss the cruelty and insufficiency of the penal system but presented new proposals on what action one can take. The current penal system ignored the fundamental causes of crime and only concerned itself with the effects of crime so Pailthorpe argued that society must learn more about the human mind and the factors producing asocial behaviour (Pailthorpe, 1933). During this period, Pailthorpe also wrote to Freud asking him if he would give her psychoanalytic treatment but he could not oblige. He instead recommended his colleague, Dr Ruth Mack Brunswick, who was also interested in Criminology (Kahr, 2018).

Some years later, in a report of the ISTD which was written in 1940, the chairman Ernest Jensen stated:

> Pailthorpe's book *What we put in Prison* attracted notice in many countries. It was my privilege to be associated with her then in regard to these publications and immediately afterwards in the foundation of the Institute of the Scientific Treatment of Delinquency which now, ten years later, has achieved a powerful and honourable position in the esteem of

government, legal and medical professions as well as of the public. Besides its recognised function in assisting the Courts, treating delinquents and conducting research, it has become an authorised teaching body for the instruction of doctors and laymen working for the Courts and dependent organisations. Its seed is germinating here and in distant lands.

(A62/1/129)

What was innovative about Pailthorpe's work for this Institute was that it gave rise to a separate brand of criminological theory with a concern for the clinical exploration of the individual personality. It sought to cure delinquents through therapy and not punishment. It originally only treated delinquent and criminal patients through psychoanalytic psychotherapy. Although Pailthorpe was intimately linked with the Institute when it first opened, all active connections ceased after she met Mednikoff in 1935. However, she remained a Vice President of the Institute until her death.

4 Further (ethnocultural-oriented) research in Africa

In early 1934, Pailthorpe was invited to Kenya by the Kenyan Government to study the increase of crime among Africans. It was also a chance for her to extend her research and look at the social problem of crime in less developed countries. This visit to Kenya coincided with an attempt by the local Government to make effective the new Juvenile Offenders Ordinance by the establishment of places of detention and later, when means permitted, of industrial schools so that the younger people would be independent from the adult criminals and be given other opportunities in life. Pailthorpe was asked to visit several prisons as well as state and private institutions. She was convinced that similar investigations to those she undertook in Britain could be carried out in Kenya with good results and was quoted as stating that "even with its mixed races Kenya offers vast scope for investigation and reforms in the handling of her criminals, and there is no reason why this Colony should not head the procession of a world-wide reform" (Author Unknown, 1934). Pailthorpe directed her research towards finding a balance between purposeless punishment and compassionate justice and formed part of the Committee of the Kenya Society for the Study of Race Improvement.

Following her stay in Kenya, Pailthorpe went to Durban in South Africa and in a speech which was broadcast all over the country on 12 September 1934, Pailthorpe spoke of the benefits of South Africa sending juvenile offenders to the Education Department. She called for the establishment of a clinic where treatment would be given to the physical and psychological state of asocial people. In her speech, Pailthorpe described Africa's chance to lead the world and ended it by saying:

> I feel that Africa has an opportunity to bring in a new civilisation built on surer foundations than the old. Her problems are acute and complicated. Is she going to deal with them courageously by the free use of research and scientific methods, or is she going to trail along using the old methods of force and bring sentimentalism, and so follow in the wake of Europe together? The eyes of the world will be upon Africa if she answers to this call, and starts out to build up, along newlines, a new civilisation. In conclusion, may I say I have fallen in love with your country; not only

DOI: 10.4324/9781003427032-5

because of its beauty, but also on account of this very opportunity, that of blazing a new trail in social organisation.

(A62 /1/029, 12 September 1934)

After her work in South Africa, Pailthorpe returned to England at the end of 1934.

5 The influences of psychoanalysis and psychiatry on Surrealism

The interest in dreams has ancient roots, but a decisive period for the development of knowledge about it was between 1860 and 1896, when research on this topic led to the discovery of almost all of the concepts that would later be found in the work of Sigmund Freud. In 1896, when Freud began his own "self-analysis" (as he defined it in his letters to Wilhelm Fliess), it was based mainly on the analysis of his own dreams (Anzieu, 1975). Subsequently, in 1901, after his patient Ida Bauer had left treatment, "Freud concluded that the case would be perfect for extending his theory of dreams into the realm of psychopathology. By analysis of this young hysteric's dreams, Freud promised to expose the unconscious underpinnings of her illness" (Makari, 1997, p. 1072).

According to the Viennese master, dreams were the manifestations of the primary process, and through the study of the dream work it was possible to explore the unconscious: "a type of thinking which is essentially non-verbal [but rather figurative and worked in images] and is, therefore, of necessity falsified by being put into words" (Rycroft, 1975, p. 155). To know more about dreams and the unconscious—since daylight thinking was of no use in that shady realm—Freud developed the method of the analyst's free-floating (evenly suspended) attention vs the patient's free associations. Freud also realised that there were elements (equal for everyone) to which patients could not associate. He came to believe that those elements were symbols, the result of a primary process that—through displacement—manages to overcome dream censorship and to discharge psychic tension. Faced with a multitude of symbols, some of which were universal, he individuated a limited number of symbolised elements: sensations, parts of the body, and primary objects (Freud, 1899).

Dreams were also fundamental to Carl G. Jung's self-analysis (see Jung, 1913–1930, 1961), which began on 12 December 1913 and continued until 1919. Indeed, it could be said that "at every crisis period in his eventful life, a dream or a vision provided essential sources for furthering a solution" (Fordham, 1978). As a young psychiatrist at Burghölzli, Jung undertook some experimental research on the word association task (see Jung, 1906). Whereas at the start of his studies, his interest was aimed at the traumatic

DOI: 10.4324/9781003427032-6

memories described by Pierre Janet (1890) as subconscious fixed ideas and the source of dissociations—so named by Janet—memories split off from consciousness (Bacciagaluppi, 2017),[1] Jung later expanded on the connection to the traumatic memories of which Freud spoke (Breuer & Freud, 1892–1895; Freud, 1896a, 1896b, 1896c). It was then that Jung gained interest in psychoanalysis.

Jung's self-analysis consisted of liberating and allowing the emergence of unconscious fantasies in the conscious mind—which must actively co-operate in order to understand symbols and make them a living experience. To achieve this aim, he resorted to techniques of introversion that can be related to the method known as "active imagination" (Jung, 1936; see also Swan, 2008). This involved either telling himself a story and writing down everything that came to his mind in relation to that story; or writing down and drawing or painting every visual expression of the Self that occurred in the dream that he could recall upon awakening. Parenthetically, according to Jung, the manifest content of the dream does not conceal a latent content: it is a representation, in symbolic form, of the internal world (structures and unconscious processes, both archetypal and personal) of the dreamer, so that "The dream is a little hidden door in the innermost and most secret recesses of the soul" (Jung, 1934, p. 144). This view of the symbol as a bridge between the conscious and unconscious, and that of the dream as something that is revealing more than concealing refers to the Freudian assumption that every symbolisation in a dream would always be defensive. Today, this viewpoint is shared by most psychoanalytic theorists (Mertens, 1999, 2000), and Jung, himself, was the first to indicate this path. Such a distinction is due to the fact that contemporary theorists conceptualised symbolisation as a psychic mechanism that implicates the processes of displacement, condensation, and plastic representation.

However today, compared to Freudian theory, the processes of displacement and condensation are considered antithetical: while through the first—better conceptualised as "substitution"—the information-processing is deferred, through the second—better conceptualised as "overlap"—the information-processing is accelerated. It follows that the mere process of displacement/substitution constitutes a pure defense operation. Among the psychoanalysts who thought that the dream is not a disguise but an expression of the dreamer's inner reality, there was Marion Milner (Stefana, 2018, 2023). Interestingly, towards the end of the 1930s, she visited an exhibition of paintings by Grace Pailthorpe and Reuben Mednikoff (Maclagan, 1992), and subsequently was shocked to discover, almost by chance, that sometimes it is possible to make sketches or drawings, allowing the eye and hand to be free to do exactly what they wish, without consciously seeking a preordained result, without any inclination to draw "something" (Milner, 1950; Stefana & Gamba, 2018; Stefana, 2023).

As seen through the discussion on Jung's self-analysis, one can infer that, for the Swiss psychiatrist, drawings are useful methods of graphically representing the nonverbal symbolic images—or rather, the best possible representation—of one's own (relatively unknown) internal world. Here, it should be noted that according to Jung (1921) the image "is a condensed expression of the psychic situation as a whole (…), an expression of the unconscious as well as the conscious situation of the moment. The interpretation of its meaning, therefore, can start neither from the conscious alone nor from the unconscious alone, but only from their reciprocal relationship" (pp. 613–614).

Such techniques, derived from self-analysis, were adopted by Jung even in his clinical work with patients:

But why do I encourage patients, when they arrive at a certain stage in their development, to express themselves by means of brush, pencil or pen at all?

(Jung, 1929, p. 48)

[Here the aim is the same as for the dreams (i.e., to produce a stimulus)]:

The creative activity of imagination frees man from his bondage to the "nothing but" [nichts als] and raises him to the status of one who plays … . My aim is to bring about a psychic state in which my patient begins to experiment with his own nature—a state of fluidity, change, and growth where nothing is eternally fixed and hopelessly petrified.

(Jung, 1929, p. 46)

During the patient's activity, the therapist's job is to avoid interfering and provide emotional holding/sustaining rather than actively intervening.

From this journey into his unconscious, Jung drew the notions of Anima, Self and individuation. He also experimented with the collective unconscious and the archetypes. The methods he used for this journey were the active imagination, the dream's amplification, the drawings and the paintings of unconscious images—methods that later became therapeutic. Therefore, we can say that it was a "creative illness" (Ellenberger, 1970, p. 672) transformed into therapeutic methodology; an unsurprising fact if we consider that "every theoretical or creative elaboration always represents the painstaking result of the introspective analysis of its author" (Carotenuto, 2007, p. 84).

In the second half of the 1920s, Melanie Klein (1926, 1927, 1929), one of the first to treat children through psychoanalysis, started to consider their playing and their drawings as an equivalent of the dreams of adults, that is, a symbolic reproduction of fantasies, desires and experiences, a spontaneous, continuous and unaware representative activity of unconscious mental content (such a view of the dream underlies the idea of a continuous stream of unconscious contents that accompanies every subject's activity). Klein pointed out that what children express in play can be understood in its totality only if we use the method elaborated by Freud for revealing the content of one's dreams. It is essential to keep in mind that to fully understand the material brought by the patient during the whole session—material which includes but is not limited to children's play—Klein takes into account not only the symbolism, which is deemed as only a part of it, but also all the means of representation, the mechanisms employed in dream-work, and the interconnection of all phenomena. Klein realised that children often represent in their play or their drawings that which had appeared in a dream and which had been described in a previous session; in this case, the play activity and the drawing mostly provide associations to their dreams. Such repetitions in different forms of the same material—or better, the repetition of the same material using different media such as the narration of the dream, toys, drawings, etc.—allow the analyst to interpret each individual phenomenon and reconnect it to the unconscious and the analytic situation. It is clear that:

> If we examine these means rather more closely—take, for instance, drawing (...)—we shall see that their object is to collect material in some other way than that of association according to rule, and that it is above all important with children to set their phantasy free and to induce them to phantasy.
>
> (Klein, 1927, p. 347)

Another meaningful contribution, of a more general cultural order, was offered by Surrealism, an artistic movement born in France in the 1920s which had recognisable elements of continuation with Dadaism (in that Surrealism attempted to put some order into Dadaism's radical disorder), primarily the exaltation of non-sense and irrationality, the wide use of mechanisms of the unconscious (psychic automatism) and of randomness. Surrealism promoted the social and creative aim of liberating mankind from a positivistic, rational, and bourgeois perspective with the purpose of encompassing a wider reality, inclusive of the unconscious dimension. The sur-reality resided in attributing to dream-work the same quality of presence, solidity, and definiteness typically attributed to external reality. The compelling influence of Freud's (1899) *The Interpretation of Dreams* is noticeable here, to such an extent that, according to René Magritte (1938), "Surrealism demands for our waking life a freedom comparable to the one we enjoy when we dream" (p. 104). The definition of the surrealist movement is provided in the *Manifeste Du Surréalisme*, where we read:

> Psychic automatism in its pure state, is the proposal to express—verbally, and by means of the written word, or in any other manner—the actual functioning of thought. It is dictated by thought, in the absence of any control exercised by reason, exempt from any aesthetic or moral concern.

> (...) Surrealism is based on the belief in a superior reality of certain forms of previously neglected associations, in the omnipotence of dream, in the disinterested play of thought. It tends to ruin once and for all, all other

psychic mechanisms and to be a substitute itself for them in solving all the principal problems of life.

(Breton, 1924, p. 26)

On an aesthetic level, the means used for liberation are automatic writing, written improvisation, and mediumistic communications; while from a pictorial point of view the means are automatism, editing, and frottage, or rather, "the rubbing by pencil of a rough surface to produce random patterns" (Chilvers & Glaves-Smith, 2009, p. 609). According to Breton, Surrealism's essential discovery lies in "the pen that flows in order to write and the pencil that runs in order to draw *spin* an infinitely precious substance" (Breton, 1941, p. 68, italic in original).

Although some distinctive signs of Breton's paternity are evident in the conceptualisation of the psychic automatism, alongside his mythical love affair with Freudian psychoanalysis (he publicly acknowledged the influence of the technique of "free association"), it is possible to identify further indebtedness toward other disciplines of the mind that lay the foundations for Surrealism (see for example Becker, 2000; Chevrier, 2007; Esman, 2011; Haan et al., 2012; Kaplan, 1989; Rabaté, 2003). Among the "researchers of the mind," the clinical use of automatism was first described in the mid-nineteenth century by the French neurologist and psychiatrist Jules Baillarger who "asked his patients to write down any thought that was coming to their minds" (Haan et al., 2012, p. 3835). Later, the concept was further explored by the most influential neurologist of the 1800s, Jean-Martin Charcot, and then more deeply by Joseph Babinski Janet (a French neurologist), Pierre Janet (a French psychologist and neurologist) and Frederic Myers (a British poet, classicist, philologist, and a founder of the Society for Psychical Research). Janet in particular had an unspoken key role.

As Philippe Soupault (1980), a friend and colleague of the leader of the surrealist movement, revealed in an interview, he was always very surprised about Breton's systematic failure to publicly acknowledge the influence of Janet. Janet's doctoral thesis, *L'automatisme psychologique* (1889) was read and re-read by Breton and Soupault in 1919 and was of special inspiration for the creation of their work *Les Champs magnétiques* (1920) through which they discovered—or better, experienced firsthand—how they could enhance access to their imagination through the liberation of a fluent and unbounded automatism of the mind (Bacopoulos-Viau, 2012). Theirs was the first attempt by members of the French Surrealist movement to systematically use automatic writing: they put down any thought coming to their mind in sentences or part of sentences that then were completed by the other one. They considered *Les Champs magnétiques* as "the first purely Surrealist work" (Breton, 1924, p. 35). But it was the automatic writing described by Janet that was the solution to their problem of poetry (whose central aspect is fusing feeling and thought into the formal unity of a work of art [Read et al., 1939]). During their early days of research, Breton made Soupault see that

... the mind disengaged from all critical pressure and scholarly habits presented with images, not logical propositions' and he told me that if we agreed to adopt what the psychiatrist Pierre Janet had called automatic writing, we might produce texts which enable us to describe an unexplored universe.

(Soupault, 1967, pp. 664–665; see also 1968, pp. 3–6)

With regard to Janet's contribution, in the introduction to his thesis he maintained that:

It is human activity in its simplest and most rudimentary forms that will be the object of this study. This elementary activity, whether noted in animals or studied in man by psychiatrists, has been designated by a name that is important to maintain – that of automatic activity.

(Janet, 1889, pp. 1–2)

Janet explained that the term "automatic" refers to a movement with two characteristics: (a) it is spontaneous because it moves itself and does not need an impulse and (b) the movement is regular and operating in a predictable, determined way. When defining "psychological automatism," Janet stated:

We believe that one can accept simultaneously both automatism and consciousness and thereby give satisfaction to those who note in humans an elementary form of activity as completely determined as an automaton and to those who want to conserve for humans, in their simplest actions, consciousness and sensibility. In other words, it does not seem to us that in a living being the activity that manifests on the outside through movement can be separated from a certain kind of intelligence and from the consciousness that accompanies it inside, *and our goal is not only to demonstrate that there is a human activity that merits the name of automatic, but also that it is legitimate to call it a psychological automatism.*

(Janet, 1889, pp. 2–3, italics in original)

Janet's work was based on detailed studies of a number of hysterical patients under various conditions of experimental hypnotism. It describes psychological phenomena observed in hysteria. Janet stated that in psychological automatism, consciousness is not connected to personal perception and lacks the personality's sense of self. This consciousness exists at a subconscious level. Thus, Janet was the first person to introduce the term "subconscious" and the concept of the existence of consciousness outside of personal awareness as he differentiated between various levels of consciousness (Van der Hart et al., 1989).

As was also the case with Freud, Charcot's teachings on symptoms of hysteria formed the basis of Janet's early theories. Janet's *L'automatisme psychologique* brought together a variety of abnormal mental states that he divided into total and partial automatisms. The former implies that the mind is completely dominated by a reproduction of past experiences and the latter occurs when part of the personality is split from awareness and following its own psychological existence. Janet believed that psychological automatism is the result of dissociation between behaviour and consciousness and that its study could lead to a new grasp of the relation between the conscious and the subconscious. According to him, patients suffering from hysteria exhibit psychological automatism in extreme degrees. He discovered that there were many mental activities occurring independently of the patient's consciousness and employed automatic writing and hypnosis—which in his view were mere experimental tools for uncovering the presence of a secondary consciousness— to best identify the traumatic origins of these mental activities and explore the nature of automatism (Van der Hart et al., 1989). However, in doing so, Janet also pathologised automatism (Bacopoulos-Viau, 2012).

Janet showed that under hypnosis, two sets of psychological manifestations can be elicited: on one side are the "roles" played by the subject in order to please the hypnotist, on the other side is the unknown personality, which can manifest itself spontaneously, particularly as a return to childhood (Ellenberger, 1970). Janet's therapeutic method involved him placing a pencil in the hand of a patient and keeping the patient's attention elsewhere. The patient would, in turn, start to write things of which he was not aware and elicit large fragments of subconscious material. In his method, Janet examined patients without there being any other witnesses in the room, kept an exact record of everything they said or did, and would also scrutinise the patient's life history and past treatments.

Janet contended that certain symptoms in a patient can be related to the existence of subconscious fixed ideas and show their origin in traumatic events of the past. He believed that memories had to be traced back to the patient's first significant traumatic event. Janet utilised a variety of visual imaging techniques to bring traumatic memories to light, including dream production, direct hypnosis, automatic writing, and automatic talking. The latter was the nearest approach to Freud's technique of free association, but Janet anticipated that his Viennese colleague would make use of automatic talking with his patient, Madame D., in 1892.

Janet's works were the intermediary between Charcot on the one hand and Freud on the other. His views on the treatment of hysteria went out of fashion when hypnosis fell into disrepute. This retreat from hypnosis was due to the publication and popularity of Freud's early psychoanalytic studies. Janet's work was neglected in favour of the acceptance of Freud's psychoanalytic observations and although Freud had initially acknowledged Janet's research, he later became critical of it (Ellenberger, 1970). Furthermore, Janet's report on psychoanalysis at the London Congress in 1913, where he claimed priority for the theory of subconscious fixed ideas that are related to intrusions of some dissociated emotion, thought, sensory perception or movement, resulted in Ernest Jones accusing him of dishonesty and asserting that Freud's discoveries owed nothing to Janet (Jones, 1914–15). However, today it is recognised that Janet's and Freud's legacies are not incompatible. On the contrary, a meeting between them could generate new theoretical and clinical insights (Cassullo, 2019).

Pailthorpe's writings suggest that she used hypnosis in her practice and this was probably because of her training with Jones in the 1920s and initial acceptance of Freudian theory (she eventually rejected the Freudian method of conducting analysis). Still, despite her association with Jones, Pailthorpe's reference to automatism when she met Reuben Mednikoff in 1935 suggests that she had discovered the concept through Janet years before she encountered Surrealist theory. It was in other words only after meeting Mednikoff, that she associated automatism specifically with Bretonian Surrealism. As we shall see, Pailthorpe and Mednikoff made extensive use of such automatic drawing, whose discovery of this type of drawings was consistent with what the psychoanalyst Herbert Silberer (1909) described as a "functional phenomenon" (p. 200), that is, the phenomenon by which, in dream images, it is the emotional state of the dreamer that is represented, and not the content of thought.

Note

1 Jung overlapped these with the emotionally charged complex of representations identified by the German psychologist Theodor Ziehen through the word association test invented by the English statistician, psychologist, and naturalist Francis Galton.

6   The relationship between psychoanalysis and art

Through Freud's teachings, psychoanalysis aimed at providing the basis for a *Weltanschauung* (worldview). A form of "applied" psychoanalysis was juxtaposed with clinical psychoanalysis. This was mostly applied and explored through the arts such as literature, poetry, music, and painting. Freud himself was committed to making use of the psychoanalytic method in investigating works of art. When doing so, he adopted two different methods: the "archaeological" method where he attempted to decipher the latent content of the works in question (see Freud, 1906), and the "psycho-biographic" method in which the biography of the artist served as the starting point for interpretation (see Freud, 1910). However, Freud himself recognised that a psychoanalytic investigation into the essence of artistic creation has its limitations even though what most interested the Viennese Master was the psychology of the artist, not the creative process that led to the creation of artistic work. Thus, a new form of research was born where psychoanalysis looked for extra-analytical confirmations of clinical insights and theoretical constructs in works of art rather than solely adopting an interpretive position. As Freud firmly believed, poets and artists in general were seen as valuable allies who had an in-depth knowledge of the human spirit and were able (as opposed to other mortals) to draw from sources inaccessible to "science." This is why the precious legacy of these poets and artists (their artistic creations) must be carefully considered (Freud, 1906). One only has to examine the role of Sophocles' *Oedipus Rex* on the conceptualisation of the oedipal triangulation, a mainstay of Freudian psychoanalysis, to recognise the impact of this new current of research on psychoanalysis.

However, the Freudian point of view on art is beyond the scope of this biography on Pailthorpe (Glover, 2009; Blum, 2017). What must be acknowledged is that Freud (1929) saw talent and artistic skills as closely related to the sublimation of inhibited sexual drives (libido). In this way, art was a substitute for satisfaction, an illusion able to counteract the harshness of life. The artist is considered to be a neurotic who shows artistic creativity (Freud, 1913). Nonetheless, Freud never came to a definitive theoretical position and never fully resolved the issue of art and artist.

DOI: 10.4324/9781003427032-7

Freud believed that relinquishing the object forms the basis for sublimation and artistic creation. This would lead to the possibility of having an aesthetic experience—endowed with specific emotions—developing out of the ability of the Ego to cope with the effort of grieving. The work of art whose form expresses the deepest of unconscious emotions is the result of this unconscious processing of conflicts with the principle of reality. However, it was Melanie Klein who more fully did justice to Freud's intuition in her theories on the paranoid-schizoid and depressive positions, which highlighted the role of intra-psychic fantasy and reparation.

Though Freud stated that the child's first relationship with the world is narcissistic, Klein claimed that the child has a relationship with the object from the start. Yet this bond is partial in the sense that the child initially connects to the breast, a partial object (which might also be considered the first aesthetic object, at least in those moments when the breast has become non-essential such as when the baby's basic needs are satisfied, thus transcending its biological and psychological functions). Klein called this configuration of the child's relationship with the partial object the paranoid-schizoid position, in which the new-born uses primitive defence mechanisms (splitting, denial, projection, and introjection) to defend himself/herself against the anxiety aroused by the fantasy that the persecutory object (unpleasant sensations, such as hunger) annihilates the self. When the infant is about five or six months, he starts to recognise his mother as a whole being, no longer partial (just a breast). This leads him to fear any damage he may have caused to the beloved object through his/her own destructive impulses and greed. Since the anxiety experienced is predominantly depressive, one can conclude that the passage from a paranoid-schizoid position to a depressive one has been initiated upon achieving this perception of the whole object (the mother as an entire being). At the same time, the child is consumed by guilt and a burning desire to preserve the object and repair the damage. This propensity to repair will continue to play a key role in the development of the processes of sublimation and in the building of relationships with others throughout the child's life (Klein, 1959).

Klein (1929) maintained that artistic creativity is linked to the concept of reparation, as depressive feelings mobilise extreme creative and reconstructive impulses. Though the process of creating art seems to have initially belonged to the depressive position; Klein later (e.g., 1958, 1960) specified that integration of the paranoid-schizoid and depressive positions is required for the success of the creative process. This integration is critical for a more balanced personality structure.

Clearly, it is within this historical and theoretical framework (when psychoanalysis begins to consider the issues related to the creative processes and not simply the results of artistic production, something which was previously ignored in the early twentieth century) that we see the original contribution of Pailthorpe. Moreover, though no date was recorded, Pailthorpe even extended her research to ethics and birth control (A62/1/008) (Figures 6.1–6.6).

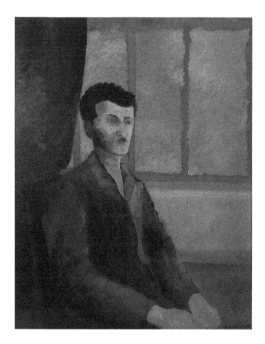

Figure 6.1 Portrait of Reuben Mednikoff by Grace Pailthorpe which included the attached note: My compulsion for snatching TM's likeness, even without glasses and in the dark, strikes me as important. Feel it has something to do with castration. If I can get his likeness—well! then he is intact (1935).

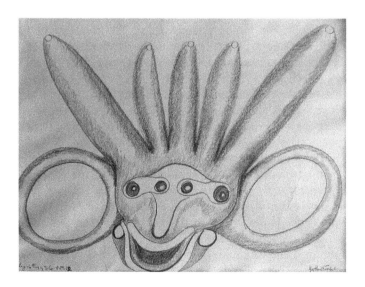

Figure 6.2 Drawing by Grace Pailthorpe (16 July 1936).

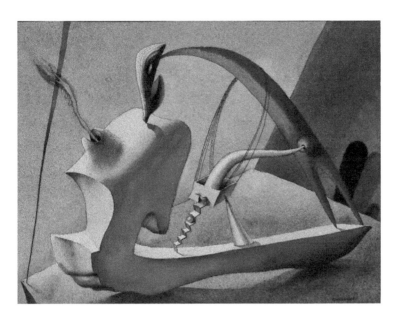

Figure 6.3 The Stairway to Paradise by Reuben Mednikoff (1936).

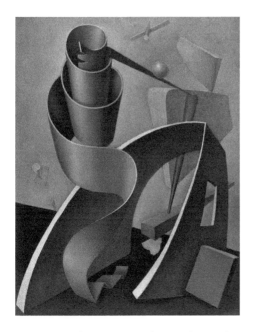

Figure 6.4 The Anatomy of Space by Reuben Mednikoff (1936).

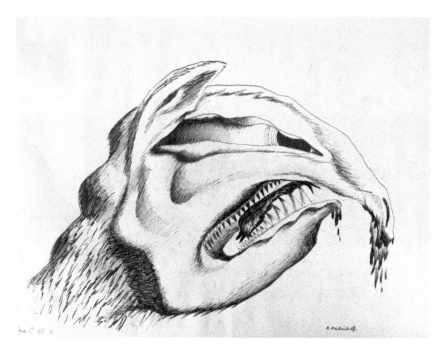

Figure 6.5 Drawing by Reuben Mednikoff (1940).

Year	Events
1883	Grace Winifred Pailthorpe born July 29th in St Leonard's-on-Sea (Sussex).
1908	Started studying medicine at the London (Royal Free Hospital) School of Medicine for Women.
1912	Went to the University of Durham's College of Medicine in Newcastle.
1914	Qualified as Bachelor of Medicine and of Surgery (University of Durham) Bachelor.
1915	Started working as a British army surgeon with the Bromley-Martin Hospital Unit in the Haute-Marne District (France).
1916	Worked as a surgeon in Salonika in the Royal Army Medical Corps of the British Committee of the French Red Cross.
1917	Set up the 'Amiens Club' in Amiens in France which served as a place of refuge for the soldiers.
1919-21	Worked as a general physician and a district medical officer in the Youanmi gold mine area (Australia).
1921-22	Travelled to Honolulu, Vancouver and New York with a friend.
	Returned to England.
	Started her study on offenders at Birmingham Prison and solely female offenders at Holloway prison.
1923	Started her psychoanalytic training at the British Institute [Analyst: Ernest Jones].
	Qualified as a psychoanalyst.
	Published *Mental tests for delinquents, and mental conflict as a cause of delinquency*, co-authored by Maurice Hamblin Smith.
1924	Specialised in psychological medicine at Holloway prison.
	Attended the Eight International Psychoanalytic Congress in Salzburg.
1925	Attended the Ninth International Psychoanalytic Congress in Bad Homburg.
	Graduated as a medical doctor (University of Durham).
1927	Finished her study of the women at Holloway prison.
	Started writing *Studies in the psychology of delinquency*.
1929	Published her review of R. G. Gordon's *Autolycus or the future for miscreant youth*
1930	Completed her analysis with Ernest Jones.
1931	Setup the Association for the Scientific Treatment of Criminals.
1932	Publication of *Studies in the psychology of delinquency.*
	Publication of *What we put in prison.*
1933	Opened and started working at the Psychopathic Clinic (was eventually called the Portman Clinic).
1934	Went to Kenya (Africa) –invited by the Kenyan Government –to study the increase in crime.
	Went to Durban (South Africa) to give a talk on the benefits of sending juvenile offenders to the Education Department on a nationwide radio station.
1935	Met and started her collaboration with Reuben Mednikoff.
1936	Participated in the International Surrealist exhibition at the New Burlington Galleries (London).
1938	Produced the Birth Trauma Series and gave a lecture on it at the British Psychoanalytical Society.
1939	Exhibited (the first joint exhibition with Mednikoff) at the Guggenheim Jeune Gallery (London).
	Publication of "The scientific aspect of Surrealism" in the December issue of the *London Bulletin*.
1940	Moved to New York (USA) with the assistance of a grant from the William C Whitney Foundation.
1941	Moved to Berkeley, California (USA).
	Joint exhibition at the 1st Exhibition of British, Canadian and American Contemporary Art at the American British Art Center (New York).
	Publication of "Deflection of energy as a result of birth trauma and its bearing upon character formation".
	Publication of "Primary processes of the infantile mind demonstrated through the analysis of a prose-poem".
1942	Went to the Rocky Mountains (British Columbia, Canada) and later moved to Vancouver (Canada).
	Started working at the provincial psychiatric hospital (later Riverview Hospital).
1943	Stopped working at the provincial psychiatric hospital.
	Founded the Association for the Scientific Treatment of Delinquency.
1944	Gave talks on Surrealism at the Vancouver Art Gallery and on the Canadian Broadcasting Commission.
	Joint exhibition (with Mednikoff) at the Vancouver Art Gallery.
1946	Returned to London, then bought and moved to a house in Sussex.
	Withdrew from public life and started working as an analyst in private practice.
1948-52	Worked as a consultant at the Portman Clinic, where led an art therapy group.
1951	Exhibited her art in an exhibition at the Artists House Exhibition in London.
1950s	Established (with Mednikoff) the first art therapy school in Dorking (Surrey, England).
1960s	Turned to Eastern mysticism.
1969	Held an exhibition of her art in the private home of Mr and Mrs Gwilym Morgan in Hastings, East Sussex.
1971	Died on July 21st.

Figure 6.6 Grace Pailthorpe, timeline.

7   Meeting Reuben Mednikoff and the start of their research project

On 21 February 1935, Pailthorpe met Reuben Mednikoff (born in London on 2 June 1906), a commercial artist and poet who was familiar with psycho-analytic principles, at a party which was given by a mutual friend, Victor B. Neuburg. Each showed an immediate interest in the other's work. Indeed, a month later Pailthorpe went to Mednikoff's flat to see his drawings and paintings. It was on this occasion when Mednikoff introduced Pailthorpe to Surrealist automatism and encouraged her to produce her own automatic writing and drawing. This encounter inspired Pailthorpe into further research of the use of art as a means of exploring the unconscious because she

> felt that there must be somewhere a quicker way to the deeper layers of the unconscious than by the long-drawn-out couch method, and I had a feeling that it was through art. At any rate it should be used in conjunction. R.M.'s quick understanding of the use and interpretation of symbols made him seem to me as probably the most suitable colleague for the research.
> (Pailthorpe, A62/1/019)

These words show Pailthorpe's dissatisfaction with the classical Freudian technique (Freud, 1912, 1913, 1919)—probably a misrepresentation of the demanding state of deprivation of both the analyst and the patient—to which she attributed the failure of her analysis with Ernest Jones. In fact, Pailthorpe found Klein's (1923, 1926, 1927, 1929, 1932) theory and technique, with which she had probably come across through Jones or Glover, more significant and made them the basis of her work.

About three months after their first meeting, Pailthorpe and Mednikoff moved to a cottage in Cornwall to start a collaborative project which involved a series of "scientific" experiments based on her psychoanalytic interpretation of his surrealist art-works (drawings, oils, and watercolours). This research continued right until Pailthorpe's death and went through four main phases (Maclagan, 1992): from their first meeting until the end of their association with the British surrealist movement (1935–40); the period they spent in North America (1941–46); their return to London (1946–mid-1950s); the remainder of

DOI: 10.4324/9781003427032-8

Pailthorpe's life (she died in 1971). Mednikoff took a less active role in the last two phases.

Most of the couple's art exhibitions took place during the first phase of their research. More specifically, they exhibited works at: the International Surrealist Exhibition in London (1936), the Museum of Modern Art in New York (1936), Kidderminster (1936), Cambridge (1937), Gloucester (1938), Toronto (Canada, 1938), Walker Art Gallery in Liverpool (1938), Guggenheim Jeune Gallery in London (1939), London Gallery (1939), Northampton (1939), and in several galleries in Australia and New Zealand (1939). An exhibition was held in Vancouver (Canada, 1944) and another two in London (1951). Lastly, Pailthorpe showed her most recent paintings at a solo exhibition in a private house in Hastings in 1969, at the age of 85. Notably, her work was acclaimed as "the best and most truly Surrealist" by André Breton at the International Surrealist Exhibition of 1936 (Walsh and Wilson, 1998).

Together, Pailthorpe and Mednikoff devised what they named the "satiation-analysis" technique. In this technique, the analyst would give the patient food and drink before the analytic session to relieve any anxiety and would then encourage the patient "to be as free as possible and to avoid, if he or she can, a desire to alter shapes that first appear (…) to paint without caring about results (…) to be loose and free with the paint" (Pailthorpe, A62 /1/022). The analyst would never help the patient whilst painting but would make gestures of reassurance, approval, permission, and sympathy if s/he showed any sign of needing it. Both participants had to make written notes about any feelings and thoughts they may have had, and every artistic production was followed by an abundance of detailed explanations. In part, the reason for these notes was for them to be able to "go(ing) over the analytic material again and again at intervals during analysis [since it] ensures an increase in assimilation of what has come to surface before [and moreover, by doing so] each time there are added details fitted into the picture" (Pailthorpe, A62/1/138, 1 March 1938).

Despite Pailthorpe's initial intention to make use of the conventional method in which the roles of analyst (herself) and patient (Mednikoff) were clearly delineated, the research transcended the conventional analytic boundaries and soon after they began a mutual analysis of Ferenczian (Ferenczi, 1932) flavour as there was a reversal of roles every fortnight. Their comments on their own work were part of their own self-analysis. The most striking thing is that Pailthorpe's interpretation of Mednikoff's art-works focused mainly on his fantasies towards her as a mother figure. In fact, Mednikoff often refers to Pailthorpe as the "mother-figure" in his notes, possibly because of the considerable age difference (she was 23 years his senior).

Between February and May 1938, Pailthorpe produced a series of brief written notes on the therapeutic results obtained through satiation-analysis, which give a glimpse of some aspects of her inner life.

First, she described the onset of indigestion and slight nausea as a temporary consequence of a psychological reactivation. In Pailthorpe's case, the nausea disappeared in conjunction with the fear related to touching ER-ER. This fear was abated when Pailthorpe started to paint three water-colour pictures with her own fingers, which seems to have constituted a loosening up of fear of close contact with dirt. With respect to the creative activity itself, she discloses how she always felt that if she stopped, then she would not be able to continue because in her mind, completing something must be done in the quickest way possible. The reason behind this attitude laid in the relationship with her brother Douglas: "If I was to work out a play-fantasy to its conclusion I had to act extremely quickly before D would notice and could and would upset things" (Pailthorpe, A62/1/065, February 17, 1938).

Although she still felt a certain degree of haste, the realisation of Pailthorpe's brother as a constant interpreter in her fantasy-play-life greatly alleviated that feeling. This realisation helped her to feel free from fear of attack from Douglas (and, on a more general level, from "the other") and, consequently, to release any inhibited normal aggression. This was an essential personal achievement since it allowed Pailthorpe to no longer need to be "the most tolerant person alive," as she had previously been called, because now that her unconscious hate was no longer of such proportion, she "can be more *truly* tolerant through understanding, and more naturally aggressive where necessary" (*ibid.*, italic in the original). As a further result of being freed from fear of attack, Pailthorpe become freer in reading the *International Journal of Psychoanalysis* and being less upset if she did not understand everything. Another important therapeutic result was the realisation of fears in relation to the self-punishment to the death of ED which provided an injection of life and vitality that she had not experienced for ages (Pailthorpe, A62/1/065, February 17, 1938).

Pailthorpe also reported having achieved further freedom by removing the inhibition of both writing and shading in drawing. Regarding the former, Pailthorpe had been at conflict with the thought of writing—which was the symbol for scratching—her own notes for a long time due to not wanting to re-experience an unconscious memory of not having the power to scratch. Although initially Pailthorpe used shading when drawing, she then stopped as they advanced in their new technique. By trying to use it and analysing the obstacle she faced, Pailthorpe immediately became aware of a horrific feeling that forced her to discard pencil for colours. The freedom to scratch and dig in (i.e., to cut) was achieved when the scratching paroxysm that had previously needed to be blanked out through the inability to scratch was expressed and dissipated through violent scratch motions of her pencil on paper.

Analysis also helped Pailthorpe identify with friends in trouble and her immediate need to show generosity. The identification with friends in difficulty had always been of such a morbid intensity that she felt compelled to do something despite being unable to bear their miseries—often with consequential detrimental effects on her. Furthermore, Pailthorpe maintained that she had always been aware of a slight feeling of being ill-at-ease when she had to refuse aid. Only through satiation-analysis was she able to change her "over-generous" nature to prevent self-damage through giving away what she needed. Still, at times she felt that her super-ego was sending feeble warnings. Pailthorpe linked these inner dynamics to her fears in relation to breast-feeding:

I had experienced a choking at the mother-breast, put down to an attacking breast or nipple because my mouth attacked it in sucking. The choking ended in vomiting and black-out. This was felt to be a nurse's attack because it happened while undergoing her attentions. I have found with a certain friend that she can only come out of her misery when demanding generosity (= breast-feeding) if she is attacked. That is her psychology. This demand for attack put me in the position of attacking nurse to myself, through the identification of myself with the friend. That meant I was asked to endure from myself as attacking nurse a vomiting and suffocation attack until the blacking-out point was reached. At this point I refused and eventually withdrew my generosity which led me to the brink of this catastrophe again and again. The fullness of this coming out here has made a marked change in my friendship to my quondam friend. After having for a long time held her off, i.e., partially abandoned her through self-defence on this score, I no longer need to do so for this reason. Neither am I driven to suffer in her suffering as if it were mine. Both these releases leave me with a normal attitude of being sorry for her, but of doing little for her at present because there is nothing that can be done except temporary efforts to cheer her through assauging her guilt sense for the time being. This freedom from the need for generosity, and the fear of having to attack has also made it easier for me in all my friendly relation-ships. They mean far less and are less demanding and engrossing a character.
(Pailthorpe, A62/1/065, April 15, 1938 & March 30, 1939)

On 5 May 1938, Pailthorpe (1938b) wrote some notes about birth trauma. This was a topic that further developed in her "Birth Trauma lecture." She wrote:

The birth trauma had just come through. During it there had been a blacking-out with each labour pain due to compression on the umbilical cord. This had been felt as a suffocation to death. The repetition of it again and again had accounted for the feeling that the process of death was unending. The new-born infant related its horrible experiences of being born to its previous kicking in the womb. Any reason is better than no reason. So the infant had grown up with a great fear of kicking = stretching in public as then it would be attacked. The public she must not stretch in front of, has always been a group which symbolically represented the mother. Stretching becomes linked up with public speaking amongst many other things in this way. 'Throwing one's weight about' = another form of stretching. This infant has always been inhibited in doing this. Where I have been freer than usual, it has always been with an Edward figure about. Otherwise I have been very reserved. Further this inhibition is always more marked when among women. The morning following the birth-trauma series was followed by great energy. I was up early and gardening before breakfast. Release from the fear of suffocating eternally in a process of death, which was unending, was also affected by this emergence of birth-trauma. But it was more gradual in realisation. Death now means one single unpleasant process and has lost from me 90% of its horror. Another marked release is in the matter of speaking freely what is in my mind. I have always been very diffident about 'stretching' my mind in the presence of others - particularly amongst those whom I would deem (often wrongly) my superiors in knowledge. 'Stretching' my mind would be dangerous since I would unconsciously be expecting an annihilating attack. When previously one has done so under the influence of kindly group (= kind mother) and I have expanded often to find myself appreciated, the subsequent pleasure has always felt to me as if I had had a remarkable and exhilarating breather, as if my lungs had been filled with a most bracing air. This release has only been noticed recently on reflection. I was able to meet all the critics of our work at the exhibition with cool and considered deliberation. I was unscared by criticism. It could no longer suffocate me to blacking-out.

(Pailthorpe, A65/1/065, May 5, 1938)

As the analysis progressed, it then focused on the issue of over-tolerance. While becoming more tolerant of others through understanding herself and them, a series of drawings on the birth-trauma experience (produced in May 1938) allowed the emergence of a memory of an incident in her babyhood which would have accounted for her marked degree of over-tolerance.

In the usual way I cried in my cot, when I had messed my nappy, so as to be taken out and cleaned up. This was the normal procedure. My cry simply meant 'Nurse, come and change me'. But nurse, instead of doing the usual did not take me up; and when I cried again, to tell her again, what had happened, she came and 'spoke angrily to me and pummeled me hard'. It is obvious she was too busy to attend to me then and was cross with me for insisting. But my infant mind couldn't understand. It felt it was not being understood and cried the more. The angry voice of the nurse and the pommeling was taken as punishment. Then nurse comes, probably only a minute or two later, and picks me up and proceeds to give me a bath. Here three separate agonies are inflicted upon me. She 'bites' with her hand (grips) my arm. She 'bites' (grips) with her hand my leg and she 'drowns' me, she holds me under water, she 'smothers' and 'suffocates' me. It is obvious what happened. She lets me slip from her grasp and I am ducked in the water, and she seizes me quickly by arm and leg and in so doing 'bites' me by too violent a grip in both places. The subsequent choking from inhaled water keeps me suffocating and smothered until I once more get my breath. To me at a few weeks old this experience is a terrific shock; something that must be avoided again at all costs. So over-tolerance is used as one means to this end. Should this break down then I must kill or be killed. It is interesting to note that since the re-experiencing of this frightful situation, I have become much more normal in showing much irritation when being baulked, by inefficient helpers around me. Neither do I feel any longer the fear of the intensity of my anger or my fear that I might kill.

(Pailthorpe, A62/1/065, May 17, 1938)

Other therapeutic results felt by Pailthorpe through her analysis in re-experiencing the befoulment of birth include the release from over-sensitivity regarding taste and smell, oversensitivity to cold, and fear of death from suffocation, as well as releasing all energy.

Based on the results obtained by Pailthorpe herself, the couple had a missionary faith in the therapeutic effects of such freedom which, thus, led to Pailthorpe forming a relation between unconscious wishes and infantile experiences which eventually developed into her ideas of the "trauma of birth." Birth trauma was a topic which Pailthorpe studied in depth over the years. She described her birth trauma, where she blacked-out (and felt as if she had been suffocated) during labour due to the compression on the umbilical cord.

8   The 'Birth Trauma' period

In April 1938 Pailthorpe (1938a) published details of an analysis in *The International Journal of Psycho-Analysis.* Here, through her analysis of a poem written by a patient during a period of treatment, she showed that artistic creation is inspired by stimuli linked to unconscious early memories. During artistic creation, the subject has no awareness of the fact that he is dramatising unconscious infantile material. Yet, he can still feel that what he is doing is related to an experience of an existing reality since the unconscious selects from any material available in the reality experience the sensation equivalent to suit the unconscious needs. The fundamental theoretical assumption is that every single word in each phrase (a) has its unconscious meaning and (b) is necessary for the word picture that is drawn.

During the course of the couple's research, Pailthorpe wrote:

> when, in psychoanalysis, some of the pent-up energies of repression were released, there would seem to be a natural turning towards some expression of the self through art (...). The art development helped on the analysis, the analysis helped on the art. The two, functioning together, produced greater art, greater knowledge in the science of mind.
>
> (Pailthorpe; quoted in Walsh & Wilson 1998, p. 41)

As this quote demonstrates, in their determination to analyse and explain unconscious behaviour during their experiments on themselves and one another, the couple's art was an automatic expression of conflicting images which run between the conscious and unconscious and the works they made were produced in their desire to reconcile themselves with their unconscious fears and phantasies. Their research was also primarily concerned with the recovery of their earliest, preverbal experiences. The aim of their interpretation of the automatic drawings which they produced was to uncover otherwise inaccessible (auditory, kinaesthetic, olfactory, and optical) memories, including the actual birth experience. Therefore, when painting or drawing, their use of automatism consisted of allowing their hand to wander across the surface without any interference from the conscious mind. Together, Pailthorpe and Mednikoff maintained that the resulting images would not be random or

DOI: 10.4324/9781003427032-9

meaningless, but would be guided by the unconscious mind, and not by rational thought or artistic training.

Pailthorpe's work with Mednikoff led her to trace all unconscious impulses back to their infantile roots—a perspective consistent with Freud's dream theory (1899). As she stated in an essay she wrote in April 1937, "sociologically we are all babies and ex-babies in our unconscious relationship to each other, and in our arrest in development, in so far as the unconscious is holding us back in any way. We are none of us parents, nor can be such to each other so long as the repressed unconscious is not fully brought up into consciousness" (Pailthorpe, 1935–37). Moreover, when describing their technique, Mednikoff wrote:

> Through automatic art a record of infantile experiences in historical sequence is obtained, consequently the exact order in which details appear and feelings arise in the patient during drawing are important in under-standing the 'picture' being presented by the unconscious. Through automatic art the fantasies that occurred during the infancy of the patient are revived, thus making analysis a fantasy interpretation procedure.
>
> (in Pailthorpe, 1937a)

The following year, when describing the process by which they produced their drawings and paintings in their 'Toe Dance Series,' Pailthorpe main-tained that "All the paintings are automatic. Nothing is changed or altered. There is no hesitation in their execution. The work is done in one swift flow. No time elapses between one drawing and another. No conscious interference takes place, or, if it obtrudes, it is set aside" (Pailthorpe, 1938c). The couple had a missionary faith in the therapeutic effects of such freedom which, thus, led to Pailthorpe forming a relation between unconscious wishes and infantile feelings that eventually developed into her ideas of the 'trauma of birth'.

Through her work with Mednikoff, Pailthorpe investigated how automatic birth anxiety forms the basis of later anxieties or fears—a point of view originally suggested by Rank (1924) where he said, "that the child's every anxiety consists of the anxiety at birth" (p. 20). She postulated that intrauterine ecstasy—in Rank's words, "the pleasurable intrauterine life" or "pleasurable primal state"—is interrupted by birth and repressed infantile memories affect one's behaviour. Such beliefs led her to produce the 'Birth Trauma Series' as a form of self-therapy and to allow her to uncover the earliest preverbal anxieties and phantasies—the ones which, according to Klein (1957), are revived in the transference situation as 'memories in feelings'. The paintings and drawings in the series consist of images of pregnancy and birth. They show the mind of the foetus during the pregnancy period. Pailthorpe deemed that even whilst the foetus is still in the womb, it is aware of every move and noise. The 'Birth Trauma Series' presents a complete picture of intrauterine and delivery experiences and manifests the sensations and phantasies (which are "bound up with sensations" [Isaacs, 1952, p. 91]) that a baby feels before and during birth. Moreover, the Series represents Pailthorpe's attempt to explore the origins of the images that haunt us. There is an innate conflict between love and hate, creation and destruction, possession and the expulsion of 'good' and 'bad' (Klein, 1948, 1957). Pailthorpe was adamant in her belief that birth, following the infant's experience in the womb, was an epochal event which left deep impressions and shaped personalities, attitudes, and people's behaviour. She explores this idea in the 'Birth Trauma Series.'

The works in the 'Birth Trauma Series' were produced automatically: as an image surfaced, it evoked another, and this continued until a complete set in the sequence had unfolded. There are six series and up to ten drawings and watercolours were created in each session where perinatal experiences were evoked. Pailthorpe produced each series on a different day and brighter colours were used as the series progressed. She noted the date and time when each work was completed and at times, wrote an analytic description on the reverse of the drawing or painting.

Soon after producing the series, Pailthorpe gave a lecture where she emphasised the primary processes of thought in the infantile mind as a way of understanding the sensations of the birth experience which led to the early steps in reasoning (Pailthorpe, 1938b). She asserted that the unconscious material in the Series provided a thorough depiction of birth experiences and affirmed "that mind is active and at work even at the time of birth" (ibid.). She described all of her works to the audience and specifically stated that she never set a time limit when it came to completing each series but instead stopped when the impulse to continue was exhausted. The precise date, place, and audience of the lecture are unknown (Montanaro, 2010).

At the start of her lecture, which she refers to as "an extract of a research which is now in its final stages," Pailthorpe states that she is indebted to Melanie Klein. Here, one must keep in mind that Klein (1926, 1927, 1929) considered children's drawings as an equivalent to the dreams of adults, i.e., a symbolic reproduction of fantasies, desires, and experiences, a spontaneous, continuous representative (unaware) activity of unconscious mental content. This point of view underlies the assumption of a continuous stream of unconscious content that characterises every person's activity. Klein pointed out that what children express in drawing can be fully understood only if using Freud's approach to dreams. She believed that the analysis and interpretation of the material in the drawings must take into consideration the symbolism, the means of representation, the mechanisms employed in dream-work, and the interconnection of all phenomena.

According to Klein, dreams and drawings, which are representations in graphic form of the inner world of the subject, allow the analyst to interpret each individual phenomena and reconnect it to the unconscious. Thus, if the analyst examines drawings more closely, s/he "shall see that their object is to collect material in some other way than that of association according to rule, and that it is above all important with children to set their phantasy free and to induce them to phantasy" (Klein, 1927, p. 347).

Furthermore, Klein (1935) maintained that the infant immediately forms a relationship with the object, or rather a partial-object relationship with the external world. For Klein, that partial object is the breast—which is the first aesthetic object, at least in those moments when it has become non-essential (Stefana, 2019). Such configuration of the infant's relationship with the partial object defines what Klein named the paranoid-schizoid position, in which the subject uses splitting, denial, introjection, and/or projection to defend himself against the anxiety stimulated by the fantasy that the persecutory object—that is, any somatic or visceral unpleasant sensation—annihilates the self. By the fifth or sixth month, the infant comes to recognise its mother as a whole object (the mother as an entire being). This arouses his fear that his own destructive impulses and greed could have damaged the loved object. It is through the achievement of the perception of the whole object that the infant begins to move from a paranoid–schizoid into a depressive state in the mind. In theorising the paranoid–schizoid and depressive positions, Klein highlights the role of intra-psychic fantasy and reparation (to which she linked artistic creativity; Klein, 1929). From a Kleinian point of view, it is in the first 18 months of life that the precursors of the subject's subsequent intellectual and emotional development lie. In this context, "The birth trauma is the first massive loss, the first physical separation, the cessation of being fed by the mother, the first physical loss experienced externally" (Payne, 1944, p. 607). The loss of the breasts comes later.

Following her reference to Klein, Pailthorpe describes how, due to the instability and upheaval felt, the "world is looking towards psychology as its last hope in a 'lost cause'." She states that she has "been dissatisfied for a long time with the results of psychoanalysis" (Pailthorpe, DGA, File 69), asserts that she has been engaged in the research over a period of four years, and claims that "as a result of this work, [I] have found a method by which psychoanalysis can be shortened and yet is more thorough in its exploration of the unconscious than has been hitherto possible" (ibid.).

Before describing each series, Pailthorpe says that the material:

will show how at this early date the mind of the infant sought for a reason to explain to itself the transition from the comfort of a quiescent womb to the turbulence and menacing experiences of the processes of being born and those immediately following birth. It will show some of the effects of these events on the subject's subsequent life and development.

(ibid.)

In her lecture, Pailthorpe tells the audience that her demonstration serves a double purpose as

Not only does it show in the minutest detail the working of *mind*, from the earliest possible moment, but it throws a very considerable light on the function of Art. It unfolds in detail what is already known in theory, viz. the work of the unconscious in the realm of Art.

(ibid.)

Pailthorpe and Mednikoff's research aimed at tracing the general effect of 'birth trauma' in the development of the individual, particularly in childhood. As Pailthorpe says, "the whole of a person's life is felt in terms of its very first trauma. I was realising that throughout life I had always felt limitations as a suffocation; as an impeding of the flow of life within me (...). In the case of my colleague, his first violent trauma was circumcision at eight days of age and throughout life he had reacted to all obstructions as attack on the penis" (ibid.). Pailthorpe believed that reliving the traumatic experience of birth during the analytic session had a therapeutic effect, and this was the ultimate purpose of each session:

> Previous to the emergence of the birth trauma into consciousness, an episode that had occurred at the age of three days had appeared and the fears in relation to it had been resolved. It appeared that I had been fed; but continued, in spite of this, to have a hunger-pain. This was due to indigestion and a vomiting-attack. Later, when asleep, I had dreamt that I had eaten the breast and that it was inside me: and that by this device I should never again be hungry. When the time came for the next bottle-feed, the teat, and possibly the rate at which the milk came, caused me to choke to the point of blacking-out, that is, becoming unconscious. This was registered by my infant-mind as an attack on me because I had eaten the breast. This revelation was followed by the recognition of the reasons for many aspects of my reactions to life.
>
> (Pailthorpe, 1938b)

Pailthorpe presented her images in front of the audience and, whilst discussing them, described how the dark background represented the darkness of the womb. She stated that "There is a mental assessment going on in the unconscious while in the womb. Everything is registered. The embryo or foetus is aware of every movement, jerk (...) increase in pressure (intrauterine) and sudden noise" (Pailthorpe, 1938b).

Pailthorpe believed that, during birth, the foetus is conscious of the womb's pressure and it resists leaving the warm womb due to fear. Despite this fear, the violent contractions thrust the infant into the outer world. Pailthorpe believed that these contractions are interpreted as the womb's angry retaliation at the foetus' persistent intrauterine kicking. She was convinced that at the moment of birth, the human being is brought into a world of conflict and confusion. Unlike the warmth and comfort of the amniotic fluid, the newborn feels pain at the sound of its own screams, the cutting of the umbilical cord, and the slap on its bottom following its birth.

In her Birth Trauma Series, Pailthorpe used watercolour paper when painting with watercolours because they had a slightly textured surface and were thicker and whiter than the paper she used for her drawings which were smaller and had a less durable surface. Her paintings show that she used the technique of blot drawing and sponging as a basis for her composition and to stimulate subconscious imagery. Her watercolours show that she used a sponge and applied it to the surface with different pressure based on how light or dark she wanted the image. Her use of tapping, smudging, smearing, and circular motions created different effects and textures (Montanaro, 2010).

The first series consists of seven drawings and watercolours. Pailthorpe makes a comparison between what the foetus feels inside the womb and what the infant feels once it is born. The first few paintings in this series convey the notion of fluidity and freedom as they suggest the happiness and safety that Pailthorpe feels whilst in the amniotic fluid. The first drawing has a playful and abstract quality. She uses pencil as her medium and the image consists of meandering, continuous lines, and curved and claw-like forms.

The naive quality of the first drawing in the series (also seen in many of the other works within the series) shows that Pailthorpe was a self-taught artist who had no academic training. Her scribbled forms, simple geometrical outlines, and diagrammatic compositions are features that are usually attributed to the creativity and spontaneity of children's drawings. Their unsophisticated style reflects her attempt to will childishness in her desire to regress to the stimulus Child Art provided. Generally, Pailthorpe's work in the 'Birth Trauma Series' demonstrates how she painted with the directness and innocence of a child's vision. Like a child, it is almost as if she was becoming aware of the story-telling possibilities in a picture.

Characteristics that are typical of Child Art can often be seen in Pailthorpe and Mednikoff's art and it was a topic that they frequently turned to. Their method encouraged one to be as spontaneous and childlike as one wished. Pailthorpe and Mednikoff collected children's drawings and could possibly have used them as a model for their own works. Sadly, these drawings have not come to light.

Even from the first series, Pailthorpe highlights the notion of 'birth trauma' during the process of birth as she ends this series with another very abstract pencil drawing in which there are colourless circular lines. As Pailthorpe tells us, in the seventh drawing the baby sees its expulsion from the comfort of the mother's womb as a punishment, and it is traumatised because it feels it has done something wrong. Prior to its birth, the baby was happy and safe in the amniotic fluid but it now experiences new sensations in a different environment. Thus, the small figures at the bottom right of Pailthorpe's pencil drawing reveal the process of the baby's final fading away to a complete black-out.

The focal point of the second series, which consists of six paintings, is the warmth and sensation of being inside the mother's womb. Pailthorpe's use of colour symbolism in Series 2 is seen and explained in her Birth Trauma lecture. The couple's comprehensive, unpublished 'Notes on Colour Symbolism' demonstrate their remarkably articulate theory of colour, in which each colour acted as a symbol for something. They believed that colour was therapeutic and that the unconscious refuses to work without colour (DGA, File 36, 9-10). When describing the colours of the mother's womb, Pailthorpe states that the blue, red, and green colours refer to warmth, the uterine water, the comfort of being cushioned, and body odour. She also refers to the colour blue as a symbol of the mother figure because of its strength and richness, yellow as representing the outside light, and black as the symbol of death.

Herbert Read's theories on colour symbolism make him a likely influence on the couple's 'Notes on colour symbolism' (Pailthorpe, 1935a). His work on Child Art may have been another source for their own. At the time, Read frequently wrote about the art of children in journals such as *The Listener*. For example, in his article, 'From the first stroke,' Read (1934) describes how infantile drawing "develops like a voyage of discovery; out of a sea of tangled scribbles emerge forms which the child recognises with delight as having some resemblance to the visual images of things seen which are stored in the mind" (p. 693). Just as in Read's statement, the intuitive aspect of childish doodling in Pailthorpe's drawing is conveyed by the impression of the pencil never leaving the paper but tracing and retracing marks repeatedly. In another article, 'Writing into pattern: A new way of teaching art to children,' Read (1938) stated that "The child 'naturally' prefers its own colour sensations to any extraneous standard (…) the sense of rhythm, both as linear flow and as sequence of shapes, so fully practised in pattern-making, is also carried over into the other activity. For with these two elements fully developed—rhythm and colour—we have the foundations of every kind of artistic activity" (pp. 1035–1036). Pailthorpe's own use of colour and sequence of shapes and lines in the Birth Trauma Series demonstrates that her professional relationship with Read, who attempted to publish her work in 1940, would have provided her with several opportunities to see how he presents Child Art. Another article discussing an exhibition of children's art was published a few months before Pailthorpe produced the Birth Trauma Series. In this article, Read (1938, p. 180) states:

> It is said that a short time ago the works of some of these children were sent in to an exhibition of modern painting without any indication of the artists ages; and that they were accepted. The story proves two things – that the selection committee of the exhibition were honest in their aesthetic reactions; and that there is a close resemblance between certain types of modern art and the art of children.

Pailthorpe's second series demonstrates how every colour had a specific meaning for her. In her analytic notes on the second watercolour in Series 2, she wrote:

> The blue shape is the womb and the central pale pink disc with the darker pink disc in it is my head with a mouth. The larger dark pink shape below this is my body. The yellow horse-shoe shape extending from a yellow disc below my body to my mouth is a nipple feeding me from a mother-breast. The other objects are milk (yellow), blood (brown) and faecal matter (green).
>
> (Pailthorpe, 1938b)

Pailthorpe also makes use of colour symbolism in the third watercolour. She tells us that she is safe within the blue womb, which lies within a green and black background:

Here I, the pink object on the left, am definitely and safely ensconced within the womb (blue). The dark surround, which is rhythmical and vibrating, is comforting because of its darkness. The pink body and head of myself is undifferentiated except for one feature:- the mouth. Into the mouth is going the yellow teat. The red and yellow shape to the right is a composite of the placenta and breast. The little yellow branch coming off the elongated nipple is equally the umbilical cord. I think this painting is saying, 'I wish the placenta-breast that fed me through my belly while inside mother would now feed me, inside mother, through my mouth'. It is interesting to note the directness of the unconscious in making a statement and its economy of language, for again the mouth is the only feature depicted.

(ibid.)

The final three watercolours in the second series render a more distinct image of the inside of a womb. The smiling baby in the fourth picture emphasises the unconscious pleasure experienced by the foetus, whilst the fifth painting also presents the idea of the warm sensation felt by the foetus but here the background is a bright red and the circle is blue. The foetus is smaller and there are fewer facial features. The same idea is expressed in the sixth and last painting in which the foetus glows with bright colours. There is an orange-coloured foetus held by red cords to the red placenta in a blue and brown background.

The third series illustrates the process of birth. It includes seven drawings and paintings. Jagged forms in the first few pencil drawings indicate the contractions and pressure as the baby is being squeezed out of the womb. When describing the fifth painting, Pailthorpe stated:

Here my head seems to have come through the tightest part of the canal and is about to come right outside. I am still colourless from compression but aware of a tremendous lot of light through the top of my head.

(ibid.)

On the other hand, in the sixth painting, Pailthorpe has come out of the womb and, in comparison to the previous paintings in this set, there is a change of colour in the face and body. In her analytic notes, she stated:

In this I appear to be well out. The strain of compression is removed and some degree of colour is coming back. The background is all the blood and faeces and moisture that surround me. At this moment I think I am actually aware of these through smell and warmth.

(ibid.)

The fourth series, which consists of only three pencil drawings, illustrates the 'birth trauma' itself. The series portrays the foetus kicking in the womb and there is an overall feeling of being attacked. This is exemplified in the second pencil drawing in the series where nine foetuses are either kicking or stretching. The zigzag lines indicate that she is kicking whereas the others show her stretching. The unborn or about-to-be-born infant is aware of its aggression in its spasmodic kicks and sees the 'throwing out' of the womb at birth as a punishment because labour is accompanied by compression and severe shock. As Pailthorpe stresses when describing this drawing, "Punishment is easier to bear than reasonless attack" (ibid.).

The fifth series, which includes nine paintings, shows the newborn baby's first screams. There is an image of a newborn baby being cut from the mother's umbilical cord in several of the paintings. When describing these works, Pailthorpe notes that in the fourth painting, she is being bathed in water. Her mouth is open and she is yelling. The red arrows are the painful noises in her head. The ring of red around her legs and the red arrows beneath her represent the nurse who pulls her up to wash and smack her bottom. The fifth watercolour also shows Pailthorpe being bathed. Here, bright red contrasts with pale pink and blue. The blue outline of the baby is the water (Pailthorpe, 1935a). The red band bound around her legs is the major point of pain. The red arrows coming out of her mouth suggest the sound that she is making. In the sixth painting of the fifth series, Pailthorpe's feet are bound by a red cord and indicate the fierce grip on her legs which causes pain. The baby is a bright pink. Her cries are getting quieter. In the seventh watercolour, Pailthorpe is crying a lot less. The grip of the red ring is gone. Still, as she says in her lecture, the towel and hands that rub her are rough (Pailthorpe, 1938b). The top part of the paper has a light yellow background whereas the remainder represents water.

The final series (ten paintings) illustrates Pailthorpe as a newborn baby and her first experiences with the environment around her. Pailthorpe states that she is awakening from her sleep following the birth trauma. The paintings depict her first experiences of being awake as she acknowledges the kaleidoscopic effects of the colours around her which she registers as a stored memory. The first watercolour is meant to represent Pailthorpe being carried. The blue and mauve colours around her are her cot. The blocks and two balls on the top right are all that Pailthorpe can see. She is aware of her new environment. The discomfort and molestation of the nurse no longer exist. As she writes in her analysis:

This is me. I feel I am being carried. I have a bunch of brightly coloured things in my hands. The blue and mauve around me is my cot. My posture makes me feel I am being lifted out of it. The two blue eyes and the faint outline of blocks, to the right, seem all that my eyes are seeing. My face is older than my usual baby faces and has a far-away-not-there look. I think the flowers are merely the sensation of many colours around me. (A62/1/069)

Most of the paintings in the sixth series have luminous colours and there is no use of pencil. Moreover, the image of Pailthorpe as a baby presents her as looking bigger and with clearer facial features than in the five previous series.

As seen, Pailthorpe's 'Birth Trauma Series' places the dyadic mother-infant relationship at the centre of the development of the subject's personality. The Series shows the experiential reality of intrauterine bliss and suffering. In both her analysis and lecture, Pailthorpe attributes the foetus in the uterus to the capacity to fantasise about rewards and punishments. She insinuates that perinatal events impinge on the development and experience of the infant. Indeed, both Mednikoff and Pailthorpe felt that psychoanalysis should include the recollection of birth and believed in the existence of an unconscious memory of embryonic days which persists throughout life and may determine all adult behaviour.

Pailthorpe's 'Birth Trauma Series' places the notion of the mother and the infant at the centre of the development of the personality. The Series emphasises the interpersonal relationship between the mother and child for it attempts to give a picture of life at its early stages where the baby is dependent on the mother for sustenance. However, Pailthorpe's psycho-analytical readings of her work are very much open to question and criticism. Moreover, although she remains known for her contribution to the understanding of the 'trauma of birth' within the psychoanalytic field, today, the theory of 'birth trauma' is no longer believed in along with the ideas that one can represent it or reconstruct memories.

9   The Scientific Aspect of Surrealism

By the turn of the year 1938, Pailthorpe published her article 'The Scientific Aspect of Surrealism' in the *London Bulletin* (the main journal outlet for Surrealist ideas in Britain) where she presented some of the results of her joint research-in-progress with Mednikoff.

Pailthorpe (1938–39) starts her article by stating that "Surrealism is one of the outcomes of a demand, on the part of those dissatisfied with the world, for the complete liberation of mankind from all fetters which prevent full expression" (p. 10). This full-expression is a biological necessity. Similarly, she continues, psychoanalysis strives, inter alia, "to free the psychology of the individual from internal conflict so that she or he may function freely" (ibid.). It follows that both Surrealism and psychoanalysis aim for the liberation of man, albeit through different paths. Thus, she claims that the fantasy-story that the unconscious unfolds when painting freely—or rather, surrealistically—is intelligible as there is always an underlying unconscious wish-fantasy for every painting. However, although "*the infantile fantasies underlying the pictures are not in consciousness at the time of painting or drawing*, (…) conscious interference in the painting can always be detected, since it invariably distorts the story in the fantasy-creation" (p. 12).

Pailthorpe goes further and states that the unconscious tells its story "with economy of language and with associations that convey the maximum effect. It gives only those details necessary for the complete understanding of its moods" (p. 15). So, "Not a line or detail is out of place and everything has its symbolic meaning. This also applies to colour. Every mark, shape and colour is *intended* by the unconscious and has its meaning" (ibid., italic in original). Such meaning can be retraced via a chain of associations starting from the images that emerge. Unconscious images are gradually produced because the infantile unconscious must overcome the fear of abandoning its cage which protects yet slows down or blocks progress. This is fundamental because "As long as fantasy-life, or the imaginative life, is free it learns by experience. (…) But fantasy or imagination bound by early infantile inhibitions and fears remains infantile in what it creates. (…) The infantile fantasy, as it becomes freer and experiences more as a result of that freedom, will grow increasingly more adult in character and its creations will show it" (ibid.).

DOI: 10.4324/9781003427032-10

Imagination and reason—which are based on human senses and dependent on what the subject has learned from experience—are interdependent. They are equally important for the sake of healthy emotional development. Being mentally healthy rather than, conversely, being mentally unhappy and limited or even pathological depends on the degree that each individual suffers from the inhibition of their fantasy-life or from the loss of their freedom in the use of reason. Pailthorpe ended her article by maintaining that the objective of Surrealism is the Self, and its goal is knowledge of the Self—which allows "the conscious and unconscious sides of our personality [to] merge to form a unity" (Pailthorpe, 1939).

The idea, expressed in the two previous papers (Pailthorpe, 1938a, 1938–39), according to which every word/mark has its unconscious meaning is also central in a later essay, 'Primary processes of the infantile mind demonstrated through the analysis of a prose-poem', published in the *International Journal* in 1941, in which, by means of the analysis of a prose-poem written by a patient, Pailthorpe endeavours to show the primary processes of the neonatal mind. Thought processes operate from birth, but the infant has no awareness of them as such, just as he has little or no awareness of the 'me' and 'not-me' that are present, and of the difference between his own muscular activity and the movements caused by external factors; what he experiences, instead, is a constant confusion between Self and Object.

However, the process of birth, the cataclysmic rat-a-tat of new events, the repeated experiences of new, unpleasant physical sensations due to extra-uterine life (and also, albeit to a lesser degree, to the intrauterine one; Pailthorpe, 1941b), represent a temporary deprivation of the state of perfect peace which affects the mind of the infant, performing a fundamental role in making the differentiation between me and not-me, between Self and Object, possible. More precisely, according to Pailthorpe (1941a) "An unpleasant experience is a 'not-me' happening. Through the removal of the 'not-me' experience, the 'me' becomes conscious of itself. It re-experiences something that previously it took for granted, namely, a state of peace" (p. 57). The mind, which constitutes a unit with the body, is the registering instrument of the bodily sensations, and it starts functioning as a reasoning instrument (to understand the details of sensation and experience registered) from the first 'not-me' experience. In this sense, we could say that "The human is born a scientist" (*ivi*, p. 59) from childhood; he observes all that he shows awareness of and, by means of reasoning, he reaches conclusions (for example, 'after this comes that') which may or may not be tainted by the lack of consciousness and experience of the external world but which he nonetheless utilises in his daily life.

In another article, titled 'Deflection of energy, as a result of birth trauma, and its bearing upon character formation' and published that same year in *The Psychoanalytic Review*, Pailthorpe shows how the entire quantum of energy of an infant is regulated and controlled by the construction of defences against the repetition of pre- and particularly post-natal traumas which entail (unconscious) deviations from the life force of the subject. A particularly relevant fact is that the unconscious material of the patient of the clinical case and its interpretation took place within a new form of analytic treatment in which various graphic media were used as a means of expression; such a method, according to Pailthorpe, makes it possible to manifest unconscious phantasies much more readily and with much greater richness of detail than with the classic method.

Unfortunately, this article does not provide any details about this new method or the graphic depictions produced in the course of the treatment, but only the interpretation of the latter and the theoretical conclusions which are now summarised here. All babies are born already in possession of great vital energy and their greatest need is to control their surrounding environment. Already in the womb, the foetus starts experiencing repeated moments of discomfort due, for example, to its cephalic position, or to uterine contractions, to which the foetus responds by kicking, in an attempt to return to its previous state. At the peak of compulsion, it yearns to destroy the not-me (the uterus) that is compressing and extruding it, and for a brief moment, as it exits the uterus, the infant thinks he has been successful in his efforts to destroy the not-me. But the forceful expulsion from his mother's womb, and the pain and suffering that he feels immediately after the birth are interpreted by the baby as a punishment for his kicking. The baby starts developing the impression that aggressive hatred and violent muscular and visceral activities (e.g., to kick energetically, to defecate, to cry, etc.) in the presence of discomfort (a not-me presence) entail being punished in the form of 'attack'.

Gradually, but rapidly, a vicious circle is established: when the baby feels attacked, he tries to destroy it but he then feels attacked again as a punishment. An example of this is that of the infant who, following birth, is suddenly exposed to the outside world. He feels uneasy and starts crying and struggling. Though the caregiver holds him, the former's handling feels painful for the baby's sensitive body who interprets this as an attack to which he responds with further struggle. Here, the infant is using his own energy exclusively to combat the repeated 'attacks' against him. The patient analysed by Pailthorpe, after a frantic search in his mind (and in his own, limited previous experience) of a way of keeping these recurrent assaults at bay, started using it also to contain his own (normal) instincts, "'If my kicking and anger at being thwarted or hurt is attacked by further pain, then', reasoned the infant—and how sound the reasoning was had the premises been correct, 'there is only one thing left for me to do, and that is to restrain my kicking and my anger'" (Pailthorpe, 1941b, p. 67). But even thus, since pain and discomfort manifested themselves every time he woke up, the additional feeling that he experienced was that of complete helplessness; and to tolerate such an emotionally intense situation, a further quota of vital energy needed to be diverted from the healthy channels to construct new defences.

The life of this patient was characterised by the constant struggle to maintain control over his own environment in order to avoid pain and suffering.

However, beyond the specificity of the case described here, Pailthorpe's objective was to show how energy can be shifted and become a destructive force that affects the physical and mental life of an individual, and how such negative forces are reflected in the character traits of an adult subject. This is particularly relevant because, according to Pailthorpe, the traumas suffered at birth have marked each one of us, making us somehow inhibited and guided by our unconscious. For this reason, she hoped that each child would be having treatment from a tender age and that, through the emergence of the unconscious deviations to which the life force of the patient has been subjected, analysis could lead the subject to full and unhindered use of his own potential.

10   The war years (1938–40)

A significant period in the lives of Pailthorpe and Mednikoff involves their efforts to reform the surrealist group in England after the outbreak of the second world war. During this period, there were internal tensions and factions within the English and French Surrealist groups particularly due to the Belgian Surrealist, E. L. T. Mesens, and his divisive demands following his move to England in March 1938. Following his arrival to England, Mesens, former secretary of the Brussels Palais des Beaux-Arts, replaced Penrose as the leading force in the British Surrealist group. He had played a crucial part in the early development of Belgian Surrealism, acted as a pivotal figure in relations between the Brussels and Paris groups, and had an important role in the extension of the movement to Britain in 1936.

A letter from Mesens to Penrose on 27 January, 1938 outlined the difficulties to be overcome for him to take over the London Gallery, which he had launched with Penrose the previous year. In the letter, Mesens defined the gallery's policy: to exhibit young Surrealists on the first floor and on the second, artists representing avant-garde tendencies from Fauvism to Abstraction. The primary goal of this policy was to attract well-known artists from Britain and overseas so that the second floor would not run at a loss.

Two months after sending this letter to Penrose, Mesens left his job at the Palais des Beaux-Arts in Brussels and settled in Downshire Hill in Hampstead. Because Penrose was frequently absent, Mesens took over the management of the London Gallery in April and, together with Penrose, launched the *London Gallery Bulletin* that same month. By taking over the gallery, Mesens aimed to establish a centre which could unite the activities of French, Belgian, Spanish, and English Surrealists in exhibitions and in the *London Bulletin*, as it was later renamed. The *London Bulletin* gave ample publicity to exhibitions at the Mayor Gallery, the Zwemmer Gallery, and the Guggenheim Jeune Gallery. Mesens assumed the post of the *London Bulletin*'s editor and his three successive assistant editors were Humphrey Jennings, Penrose, and George Reavey. It was published almost every month and contained many reproductions, poems, and articles. The London Gallery also operated a lending library that became a magnet for artists, poets, and writers and contributed to the development of Surrealist activities in England. In June 1938, Penrose left England for Paris

DOI: 10.4324/9781003427032-11

and then joined Lee Miller in Athens. Due to Mesens's many contacts abroad and those of Penrose in Britain, Mesens succeeded in maintaining a solid surrealist presence in London during Penrose's absence.

Meanwhile, the political atmosphere in Europe was becoming increasingly tense and repressive. In France, the Communist party was banned and many of its leaders were either imprisoned or forced into exile. Although the struggle between Republicans and Nationalists in the Spanish Civil War had begun for purely internal reasons in 1936, the conflict played a significant role in shaping Great Power politics. Pailthorpe and Mednikoff showed no interest in the Spanish Civil War, but merely retreated away from public events and into their own private world. Their art also demonstrates this, as, unlike artists such as Dalí, none of their works carry political overtones.

The Spanish Civil War profoundly influenced the two major alliances of the interwar period: that between Italy and Germany on the one hand and between Britain and France on the other. The Nationalists in Spain appealed to Germany and Italy, and the Republicans to France and the Soviet Union. Through events in Spain, ties between Germany and Italy became closer, and the French found themselves bound tightly to their British allies. Thus, the differing decisions over intervention or non-intervention clarify the conditions under which the great powers were willing to go to war. The growing threat of Germany pushed France and Britain closer together in the 1930s, and their union was the optimal and only solid hope in Europe that peace might be restored. Because Belgium feared that Germany was a menace to its security, the Belgians announced that they favoured neutrality. They overturned the 1920 military agreement to cooperate with France and reduced France's security by leaving the Franco-Belgian border unprotected. Despite this, both Britain and France expressed their determination to defend Belgium against unprovoked aggression.

Throughout this tense period, the Surrealists did not abandon their political activities and supported all the left-wing groups in the Spanish struggle except the Stalinists. Unlike so many disillusioned ex-Communists, the Surrealists never turned to the Right and Breton's next political move was to align the movement with Trotsky, with whom he established close personal ties after his visit to Mexico in 1938.

Strife within the Surrealist group in England likely began just after Breton's meeting with Leon Trotsky, which came about through Diego Rivera, at whose house Breton stayed during his visit to Mexico between April and September 1938. Breton travelled to Mexico after accepting a cultural mission from the French Ministry of Foreign Affairs to give a series of lectures on French art and literature. The reason why he was willing to give such lectures was because it would give him the opportunity to meet the exiled revolutionary Trotsky in person. As Polizzotti wrote in *Revolution of the Mind*, the Stalinists regarded Breton's visit to Mexico with evident suspicion and, before his arrival, a French Communist organisation sent a letter to the major Mexican writers and artists calling him a 'propaganda envoy from the Ministry of Foreign Affairs'. Aragon also sent a letter to the Association des écrivains et des artistes révolutionnaires (A.E.A.R.) urging the Mexican Stalinists to affect a "systematic sabotage of all Breton's activities in Mexico." Despite these attempts to discredit him, Breton was warmly received in Mexico.

Breton found in Trotsky an understanding man who believed that to maintain its revolutionary character, art must be independent of all forms of government, must refuse all orders, and follow its own process of development. Because of their shared concern for the freedom of art and their stand against social realism, this meeting resulted in the two of them collaborating and producing a new manifesto entitled *Pour un art révolutionnaire indépendant* and dated 25 July 1938. It condensed many of Trotsky and Breton's discussions on art and politics. Since Trotsky was forbidden by the Mexican government to engage in any political activities and because he believed that the manifesto should be signed by two artists, it appeared under the names of Breton and Rivera. This was only revealed after Trotsky's death in 1940.

The manifesto addressed all leftist intellectuals who refused to follow the call of Stalinism:

> We do not explain that at no time—no matter how favourable—do we feel any solidarity with the slogan "Neither Fascism nor Communism!"—a slogan for conservative and frightened philistines clinging to the remnants of a 'democratic' past. True art, art that does not rely on producing variations of already existing models but tries to express the innermost needs of man today (...) such art must be revolutionary; it must be aimed at a complete and radical revision of the social order.

The manifesto condemned both the Fascist and Stalinist regimes for repressing and destroying progressive art and condemned the decadence of bourgeois democracies. It affirmed "once again the principles of freedom in the service of the revolution," and relied on psychoanalysis 'to demonstrate that it is only by bringing the repressed elements of the human personality into harmony with the ego, and not by repressing them further, that man can be emancipated'. Freudian theory was used to illustrate the psychologically damaging effects on the artist of the conflict between his ego and the hostile environment in which he must live. Breton and Trotsky also wrote that art should be isolated from politics and demanded that, "In the realm of artistic creation, the imagination must escape from all constraint (...) To those who would urge us (...) to consent that art should submit to a discipline which we hold to be radically incompatible with its nature, we give a flat refusal, and we repeat our deliberate intention of standing by the formula complete freedom of art."

The purpose of the manifesto was to provide an alternative to all totalitarian restrictions. The final part of the manifesto included an invitation to the revolutionary artists of all nations to unite in forming a new organisation which would be called the Fédération Internationale de l'Art Révolutionnaire Indépendant (F.I.A.R.I.):

> Revolutionary, independent art should unite for the struggle against reactionary persuasion and for a loud proclamation of its right to existence. Such a campaign is the aim of the 'International Federation of Independent Revolutionary Arts' which we consider necessary to create.

Thus, the manifesto sounded a call to unite all those who had decided to "serve the revolution through the methods of art, and to defend the freedom of art against the usurpers of the revolution." Breton and Trotsky stated that:

> The aim of this appeal is to find a common ground on which may be united all revolutionary writers and artists (...) Marxists can walk hand in hand here with anarchists provided both parties uncompromisingly reject the reactionary police patrol spirit represented by Joseph Stalin (...) Every progressive tendency in art is destroyed by fascism as 'degenerate.' Every free creation is called 'fascist' by the Stalinists. Independent revolutionary art must now gather its forces for the struggle against reactionary persecution.

Ultimately, Breton and Trotsky's manifesto called for a revolutionary art that differed from art promoted and patronised in Stalinist Russia, the Fascist dictatorships, and the bourgeois democracies. As Helena Lewis says in *The Politics of Surrealism*:

> The manifesto clearly rejected the doctrine of socialist realism, as well as the reactionary bourgeois 'art for art's sake' school of aesthetics. It called upon a broad coalition of left-wing artists who had also rejected both these alternatives to come together, and specifically extended an invitation to anarchists to join the F.I.A.R.I. thus emphasizing the libertarian nature of the project.

After returning to Paris in early September 1938, Breton learned that Eluard had been writing for *Commune*, the Stalinist A.E.A.R. journal, which had tried to sabotage his Mexican visit. Aragon, who had renounced Surrealism to become a Communist party militant in 1932 which then led to the end of his relationship with Breton, was the editor of *Commune*. Because he saw this as an act of personal and political disloyalty, Breton ended his relationship with Eluard, although he was once one of Breton's closest friends and one of the original founders of the Surrealist group. The break between them ended a 20-year friendship, and, following this, the Paris correspondent of the *Partisan Review*, Sean Neill, wrote that it was "a shock that Eluard's sense of expediency has made so brilliant a poet prefer continuation of his connection with the Stalinist *Commune* to signing the F.I.A.R.I. manifesto."

Due to his split with such a greatly admired poet and much-loved man as Eluard, Breton's need to establish F.I.A.R.I. became even greater, and once he was back in Paris, Breton set about creating a French section of the Federation that had been proposed by the Trotsky-Breton manifesto. He called a meeting of Surrealists in Paris to denounce Eluard's attitude towards Stalin. So vengeful was Breton that, driven by personal friendship, other Surrealists like Man Ray, Ernst, and Georges Hugnet preferred to follow Eluard and left the Surrealist movement in October 1938. Still, a national committee, consisting of Breton, Yves Allégret, Michel Collinet, Jean Giono, Maurice Heine, Pierre Mabille, Marcel Martinet, André Masson, Henry Poulaille, Gerard Rosenthal, and Maurice Wullens, was formed and represented revolutionary art in France. Those who agreed to collaborate with the left-wing F.I.A.R.I. in response to a questionnaire forwarded by Breton included Read, Mesens, Jef Last, Francis Vian, Serge, Paul Benichou, Albert Parez, Jean-Francois Chabrun, Nadeau, Cahun, Nicolas Calas, Michel Carrouges, Robert Blin, Marcel Duhamel, Marcel Jean, Ignazio Silone, Thirion, and Henri Pastoureau.

On 9 September 1938, the English Surrealists received a handwritten copy of Ian Henderson's translated text of Trotsky and Breton's manifesto. Read was the only English person to sign up. This placed him in a different political camp to Penrose, who did not sign the manifesto because he was very close to Eluard. One can see why Mesens was inclined to sign the manifesto since, together with Magritte, Nougé, Scutenaire, and Souris, he had signed 'L'Action Immédiate.' The latter was published in the special issue of the journal *Documents 34* in June 1934. It was entitled 'Intervention Surréaliste'and it explored the conditions favourable to revolutionary activity outside the Communist Party.

The membership of Breton's committee reached nearly 60 by late September 1938 and began publishing its own bulletin, *Clé: Bulletin mensuel de la FIARI*, with Maurice Nadeau as editor. *Clé* was primarily a political journal, yet the freedom of art was one of its dominant themes. It was also as much opposed to French government policies as to Stalinism and Fascism. Although the Paris group was the most numerous and best organised, F.I.A.R.I. groups were simultaneously formed in Mexico and Buenos Aires.

A letter from Breton, addressed 'To our friends in London,' dated 21 October 1938 and translated by Maddox (a supporter of Breton), stated that the British group must define its position towards Trotskyism:

> At the moment we expected to hear of the constitution of the English section of the FIARI, Penrose informs us that you have not been able to agree on a plan of action. The question which seems to worry you most is what attitude to adopt towards the USSR.

Breton emphasised, "that to unite with all the creative forces of man, by all critical and effective means—and we do this when we take as a starting point the class struggle—is the highest task to which an artist and an intellectual, worthy of the name of revolutionary, can aspire." He wrote that "if the leaders of the proletariat had not committed errors, there would never have been Fascism either in Italy or in Germany" and as a consequence, "not to react when faced by the faults of the Third International would be tantamount to acceptance of the responsibility for its errors and its crimes." He ended the letter by writing: "We fight for the Independence of Art by the Revolution, as we fight for the Revolution by all effective means."

According to Michel Remy, in a previous exchange of letters with Breton, Penrose had defended an alliance with the Communist party to prevent any isolation in the fight against Fascism. Because of his work for the cause of the Spanish Republic, Penrose remained on good terms with the British Communist party but did not become a member. Due to his links with Paris, he became the political spokesman for the British Surrealists, but refused to allow any political disagreement to come between him and Eluard. Moreover, he could not assure Breton of the support of the British group, which tolerated a wider range of political attitudes, with some members being Communists, Marxists, or sympathisers of one shade or another. Breton refused to sanction such unorthodoxy and stressed that unity amongst the Surrealists was crucial:

> Certain Surrealists in London, it appears, hesitate. We hope that this letter will help them to dispel their fears. If this is not the case, it is obvious that they will only be surrealists in name. We are not deceived by words or labels, no more by the label 'communist' or USSR.

Breton and Trotsky's shared ideas on art and politics in their manifesto gave voice to the drift of British Surrealism away from Stalinist Marxism towards Trotskyism. *Pour un art révolutionnaire indépendant* was published in French in the *London Bulletin* in October 1938. Beneath the heading, a note to the reader states (in English):

> We reproduce here the full text of a Manifesto by Andre Breton and Diego Rivera, written during Breton's recent visit to Mexico. We hope to publish an English translation in our next number.

Sure enough, an English translation of the manifesto was published in the next issue of *London Bulletin*, which also included Pailthorpe's article on 'The Scientific Aspect of Surrealism'. Beneath the heading there is another note to the reader:

> In accordance with our promise to readers in the preceding number, we now publish the English translation of the Manifesto by Andre Breton and Diego Rivera. We print this text from a documentary point of view.[1]

By publishing the manifesto in the *London Bulletin*, the English were adhering to Breton's requests. However, despite the French attempts to make the English conform, the English group could not come to agreement due to their shock at the violently uncompromising attitude expressed in the manifesto. The note to the reader explicitly states that the manifesto is printed "from a documentary point of view" and not as a sign of allegiance. Thus, it is likely that the start of the collapse of English Surrealism as a unified movement can be dated from this period due to Breton's attempts to extract greater political commitment from the British contingent. Although there was agreement on the need to oppose Fascism in Spain, the main conflict was centred around the attitude the Surrealists should take towards the Communist parties controlled by Moscow. However, no articles on internal disagreements within Britain following the publication of Breton and Trotsky's manifesto, the expulsion of Eluard and the formation of F.I.A.R.I. were published in the *London Bulletin* at that time.

Like Breton, Read was sympathetic to Trotsky's insistence on a separation of the artist from the state. He abhorred Stalinism and saw Communism as a stifling political system. His reaction to Breton's attempts to make the English conform was printed in the first issue of *Clé* in January 1939:

Dear friend,

Today Mesens has shown me your letter and the manifesto. I hasten to say I completely agree. I have already expressed myself in that sense. Certain pages of my recent book *Poetry and Anarchism* are almost word for word those of the manifesto.
Needless to say that I am ready to adhere to the Federation which you are now forming
Affectionately yours,
Herbert Read

After visiting Eluard, Ernst, and Hugnet in Paris, who were all alienated from Breton and who also became Communists, Penrose sent a letter to Read on 27 January 1939 in which he advocated the publication of another manifesto which would "help English intellectuals to clarify their own position" and build "a group of revolutionary anarchist intellectuals with a very definite programme behind it." He concluded that "The idea of a united international surrealist activity is now a thing of the past (...) my feeling is that we should do well to soft pedal on all issues which might enfeeble even further revolutionary tendencies, some sort of unity must be attained and self-criticism which prevents this looks like a kind of neurosis, a self-destructive force."

This letter proves that the disorientation felt by artists encouraged them to form different factions. German troops were occupying Czechoslovakia from 14 January 1939 and the general consensus among the Surrealists was that neither liberty nor the creative spirit could prevail against the power of the state. This is seen in Read's article 'L'Artiste dans le monde moderne', published in *Clé* (II) in February 1939, which states:

> In our decadent society (…) art must enter into a monastic phase (…) Art must now become individualistic, even hermetic. We must renounce, as the most puerile delusion, the hope that art can ever again perform a social function (…) This is equally true in Russia and in the West. Art has become nonsense (because) it matters little whether your army is military or industrial; it is still an army and the only art appropriate for an army is the music of a military marching band.

After only two issues, *Clé* became one of the many casualties of the Second World War. Breton later commented: 'the unity necessary for the success of the F.I.A.R.I. was lacking by a great deal, so that *Clé* disappeared after its second number. Yet, this failure, at such a moment, was compounded by so many others: intellectual activity in general came to a halt because thinking men had already decided that nothing could turn back the scourge of war'. Despite its belief in the freedom of the individual and artistic expression and in the international character of culture in opposition to nationalism of any kind, F.I.A.R.I. failed to resolve the problem of how the revolutionary artist was going to function. Furthermore, apart from Maddox, Mesens, Read, and Penrose, there were no other replies from England to Breton's call to join F.I.A.R.I. Pailthorpe and Mednikoff's failure to adhere to F.I.A.R.I. also illustrates their lack of concern for political events. Additionally, although Breton made a request for Surrealists to boycott Eluard or face expulsion, Penrose remained loyal to Eluard as he was his closest friend in the movement. Possibly because he was buying art from Breton, Penrose escaped the latter's disapproval and remained on good terms with both him and Eluard.

With certainty, WWII led to the dispersal of the Surrealist group. Many artists either joined the army or left London, and galleries closed as the art market collapsed. Pailthorpe and Mednikoff left Cornwall and moved to Hertfordshire once the war was declared. Although there is no evidence as to why they moved to that specific area, Mednikoff was excluded from any military duties because of his medical history. Their move to Hertfordshire also meant they had easier access to London. At this time, the Surrealist group had already started to fragment due to the various factions within it and because the war led to the financial collapse of the art market. Moreover, in 1939, due to his work on French broadcasts for the BBC during the war, Mesens had to close the London Gallery, which hitherto had acted as a nerve centre for Surrealism in Britain. The *London Bulletin*, which had become the British Surrealist mouthpiece, also ceased publication in June 1940.

Pailthorpe and Mednikoff now tried to rescue the situation by promoting the reformation of a cohesive group and discussion of the position of Surrealism within the art world. However, their main motive may have been due to their desire to participate in as many exhibitions as possible and, to some extent, to restore the failing art market. Their plans to organise a Surrealist group exhibition at the British Art Centre at the Stafford Gallery in St James' Place in London during the months of June and July in 1940 suggest this. The couple favoured the British Art Centre over other galleries because of their existing relationship with Guggenheim. Unlike Mesens and Penrose, Pailthorpe and Mednikoff had no personal entanglement with her and were also close to Read, who was himself close to Guggenheim.

Although there is no precise date, the organisation of the intended exhibition began in early 1940. A form written by the gallery's founder and secretary, Ala Story, on 3 March 1940 stated that no work would be accepted or judged unless the artist was a member of the British Art Centre and that the gallery would also charge a commission of 33.3% on the actual price paid for any work of art sold at the exhibition. In a letter to Mednikoff dated 25 March 1940, Story suggested that the Stafford Gallery and the couple should split the percentage on sales and also halve the cost of printing the catalogue. Soon after, in a letter to Story dated 4 April 1940, Pailthorpe stressed the fact that the couple's own works were intrinsic to their research project:

> I wish to state again, as a reminder, that the conditions of sales of my works (and Mr. Mednikoff's works) are that we retain the reproduction rights, and before a painting or drawing leaves your hands that we are permitted to have colour blocks, or half-tone blocks, or line blocks (as the case may be) and photographs made. We, of course, pay for blocks and photographs.

The correspondence reveals their personal motives as, besides being determined to save the Surrealist group, they also wanted to show their art in order to generate sales so that Pailthorpe could publish her work. Moreover, the fact that they were splitting proceeds with the British Art Centre meant that they were eager to promote sales.

On 16 March 1940, Mednikoff sent invitations to various members of the Surrealist group in which he wrote that the exhibition provided the possibility "whereby the activities and works of Surrealist creators can resume, as a body, a vital contact with the public." Mednikoff continued:

> We are, therefore, taking the liberty of enclosing details of the 'British Art Centre' (which, we hope, will interest you) as only members of this group are permitted to submit works (three from each member).
>
> As your co-operation will enable us to encourage the organising of the exhibition, we would be glad if you will let us know, as soon as possible, whether you feel inclined to become an 'artist member' of the B.A.C.
>
> We are enclosing a signed 'application form' to save time; and this should be sent direct to the Stafford Gallery if you decide to join. But whether you accept or decline this opportunity, we would greatly

appreciate a postcard informing us of your decision as there is little time left for us making the necessary arrangements.

The Stafford Gallery exhibition was planned to be held between 12 June and 6 July 1940. The handwritten draft of the catalogue is headed 'An exhibition of Surrealist paintings and drawings. The first part of the catalogue was supposed to include an introduction by Read, called 'An interesting article' but no trace of this essay—if it was ever written—has survived.

After listing the names of the exhibiting artists, the draft catalogue ended with a typescript of Mednikoff and Pailthorpe's article: 'Will Surrealism survive.' In this article, they wrote that "More literature has been written on this movement by the creators themselves than has been the case with any other change in the trend of art." They claimed:

When the emotional content of a work is great it possesses power and vitality; and it maintains an active control of the onlooker's interest. If such a work is created with skill, and stirs one deeply, it is called 'immortal.' Some of the works of El Greco, Turner, Blake, Van Gogh, Picasso and numerous primitive carvings possess a high degree of affective content. It is the richness of this quality which makes them 'live'. In other words, it is the intensity with which the artist has manifested his or her deepest feelings that decides whether a work of art shall survive the varying moods and opinions of humanity.

The article ends by stating that, "Because Surrealist art gives a legitimate, or socially tolerated, outlet to the inner emotions, it, like religion, will endure; for the need of mankind for an emotional outlet is a dynamic force which will ensure its survival." This article clarifies how Pailthorpe and Mednikoff were driven by their conviction of the importance of their own work.

Artists who agreed to exhibit and are listed in the draft catalogue include: Mednikoff, Pailthorpe, Ruth Adams, Eileen Agar, Cecil Collins, William Johnstone, Rita Kernn Larsen, Len Lye, Alastair Stewart, Edith Remington, Robert Baxter, Leslie Hurry, Charles Watson, and Ithell Colquhoun. Each artist was asked to exhibit three works. Artists who refused to exhibit included F.E. McWilliam, who pointed out that he was a sculptor and not a painter and stated that he disliked the British Art Centre, and two others who signed as 'Charles' (and gave no reason) and 'Pat' (who was not keen on parting with her works).

Penrose was one of the artists whom the couple invited to exhibit, and four days later he replied:

Dear Mednikoff,

Thank you for your letter. The prospect of a surrealist exhibition in June at the Stafford Gallery is of course of great interest to me. I should certainly like to participate in it but there are certain points which I would like to elucidate first.

Since there are a good many questions that I should like to ask, would it be possible for us to meet in London if you are by any chance coming to town soon?

In order that the show should be genuinely surrealist and not dominated by the atmosphere of the B.A.C., it is essential that the choice of the artists and the exhibits should remain entirely in the hands of the surrealists. If you have been given a free hand in this way I have great hopes of this show being a success.

Have you made out a list of painters who you are inviting? If so it would interest me to know who they are. I am not sending my application for membership of the B.A.C. until I have been able to discuss these matters with you.

I shall be very glad if Dr Pailthorpe and yourself could manage to lunch with me in town. Could you let me know when you are likely to be able to come?

Yours ever
Roland Penrose

Penrose's circumspect reply suggests that he knew that the exhibition would create tension within the Surrealist group and that he feared it would not be an exclusively Surrealist exhibition. Penrose knew that the British Art Centre was not a strictly Surrealist gallery and surely feared that all sorts of artists would be allowed to exhibit. Perhaps he suspected that the motives of the couple were to make money so that they could publish their research, rather than altruistically wish to aid the reformation of the Surrealist group by organising an exhibition. In the end, Penrose must have refused to participate because his name is not listed in the catalogue draft.

Following the couple's meeting with Penrose in London, Mednikoff wrote to the members of the Surrealist group on 1 April announcing a meeting at the Barcelona restaurant in Soho:

At a meeting between Dr Pailthorpe, Roland Penrose, W Hayter and myself, it was decided that arrangements be made for a gathering of Surrealists for the purpose of planning the reforming of the Surrealist Group in England.

Dr Pailthorpe and I suggested the reforming of the group with freedom from political bias or activity as part of its constitution. As it was felt by us all that Surrealism's vital purpose would benefit considerably by the reforming of the group, it was agreed that arrangements be made for a dinner, to be followed by a discussion in which all views could be made known and a constitution formulated.

The plans for this are now in progress. The dinner will be held on Thursday, April 11th, at 7.15 pm, and the price will be 3/6 per person.

The final arrangements cannot be made until the exact number of people who will be present is known, therefore, it is essential that I am quickly notified of your intention to be present. As soon as I receive this information the address of the rendezvous will be sent to you. Because there is very little time to spare an immediate reply will be greatly appreciated.

Yours sincerely

Although there is no evidence as to which Surrealists he sent the invitation to, Mednikoff received a reply from the Birmingham group of artists. Interestingly, at the time, Surrealist activity developed mostly outside London probably because of the difficulties met by London artists due to their various political alliances, the effects of war, and the closure of the London Gallery. London was also a target for enemy attacks and very dangerous. Initially, Birmingham was seen as a provincial, Quaker city with limited opportunities for a contemporary artist. However, a group of like-minded Birmingham artists—among whom were Conroy Maddox, John Melville, and his brother Robert—overcame second-city inferiority and took on the art scene in London. As Remy says, the creation of the Birmingham group in 1935 was in part a form of reaction against the parochial nature of the city and the conservatism of its official art organisation, and thus the group maintained a spirit of artistic rebellion. Together with Maddox, John and Robert Melville, Eric Malthouse, Desmond Morris, Emmy Bridgwater, Oscar Mellor, Stephen Gilbert, and William Gear formed the nucleus of the Surrealist group in Birmingham.

According to Silvano Levy, for over half a century Maddox reiterated the view that in their haste to gather a sufficiently large number of exhibitors, the English organisers of the International Surrealist exhibition had solicited artists who were not committed to the movement:

No doubt it was possible to perceive this Surrealist imagery in a lot of paintings, but that hardly made them surrealist. There is a big difference between the imagery and the philosophy. It is easy to confuse imagery with purpose. Surrealism is concerned with expanding our definition of reality, not with producing images that are merely fantastic or nonsensical.

Melville also stated that, as far as the Birmingham trio were concerned, there was an ideological gap between them and those who had been eager to exhibit at the International Surrealist exhibition and that the Birmingham group had deliberately distanced themselves from what they regarded as less than purist tendencies. He satirically wrote: "Birmingham was at the end of the earth, but it's one of the privileges of provincials to be extremely purist, and if London was trying to make a contribution, we were not interested."

In an interview with Robert Short in 1978, Maddox stated that 'Paris was the fountainhead of surrealism' and that the Birmingham group was "concerned only with the creative source, the small Parisian sect." The Melvilles and Maddox avidly followed news of developments, quarrels, and defections among French Surrealists and this made them aware of the 'orthodoxy' of their position as 'we were always on the side of Breton'. This caused the Birmingham group to distance themselves from the arrangements initiated by Read and Penrose in England in 1936 and in his interview with Short, Maddox claimed that they 'did not join the English group until 1938 when it had undergone significant changes'. He stated that Read was to be blamed for 'the seed of destruction that was going on around 1936 and after'. On the other hand, Maddox approved of Mesens:

> When the International Surrealist exhibition ended, Surrealism in England almost disappeared. It was due to Mesens that a limited activity continued through the London Gallery with exhibitions and meetings.

Because of their protests at the 1936 International Surrealist exhibition, Maddox and the Melville brothers were conspicuously absent from all British Surrealist exhibitions. In fact, the first documented public connection of Maddox and John Melville with the Surrealist group in London was in January 1939 when they participated in the 'Living Art in England' exhibition. Pailthorpe and Mednikoff also exhibited their works there. The exhibition was organised by Mesens who emphasised that "This exhibition was intended to present a united front of the most radical moderns as an opposition to the growing decay in Europe under the pressure of the Nazi art politics and intolerant attitude of the tenets of Socialist Realism."

Like Pailthorpe and Mednikoff, the Birmingham group was not party-political. In fact, the major Birmingham Surrealists were relatively unaffected by the onset of war since they all had reserved occupations and this made them exempt from military service. In their letter to Mednikoff, Maddox and the Melville brothers wrote:

Dear Mr. Mednikoff,

We are extremely interested to hear that you are attempting to resuscitate the English Surrealist group on a non-political basis, and wish you every success. It would of course give us great pleasure to attend the meeting on April 11th, but we feel that at this stage anything we might have to say would be an unnecessary intervention and that nothing should be allowed to hinder the immediate aim of uniting Surrealists in and about London.

We take it for granted that you are not calling upon Surrealists only for the purpose of holding group exhibitions - and on the face of it there is no easy solution of the problem of how Surrealists in the provinces can usefully co-operate with the main group. All the same, we would appreciate the opportunity of meeting you at a later date, to enable us to state a case for the provinces.

Meanwhile, we hope that you will let us know the results of next Thursday's meeting, and we ask you to accept our assurance that we are always ready to do anything within our power to propagate the movement.

Yours sincerely,
Robert Melville
John Melville
Conroy Maddox

As detailed by Levy in *The scandalous eye: the Surrealism of Conroy Maddox*, a few days before the 'Living Art in England' exhibition, Maddox attended a private viewing of Pailthorpe and Mednikoff's art exhibition at the Guggenheim Jeune Gallery and was thus already familiar with their research before writing this letter. However, despite their will to eventually 'state a case for the provinces', it seems that the Birmingham group remained sceptical about the Surrealist credentials of any artists who had participated in the 1936 exhibition. Furthermore, the Birmingham group's letter to Mednikoff illustrates how the couple's plans were an attempted non-political reformation of the Surrealist group and this risked them causing another division between themselves and other members of the Surrealist group because it can be presumed that they wanted to form a faction with other non-political Surrealists.

On the other hand, Read expressed approval of the couple's efforts to reform the group in a letter written on 1 April 1940, the same day that Mednikoff issued his invitation to the Barcelona meeting:

Dear Mr. Mednikoff,

I have to go up to Leeds next week, but I hope to be back on the 11th and will if possible come to the dinner you are arranging. I think we certainly ought to meet and consider the situation and carry on some sort of activity.

Yours sincerely
Herbert Read

In particular, Ithell Colquhoun was the one who firmly supported the couple's plans for the meeting. In a handwritten letter dated 5 April 1940, she wrote:

I shall be very pleased to come to the dinner you and Dr Pailthorpe are arranging to discuss the future of Surrealism in England. As you know I am in agreement with your idea of the non-political basis of any group which may be formed.

At around this time, Penrose sent a handwritten invitation to Pailthorpe calling her to a meeting of the Surrealist group on 7 April at his house at 21 Downshire Hill at 8.30 pm. This indicates that although he was not prepared to participate in their proposed exhibition, he recognised that she was now a powerful figure and could not be marginalised or ignored.

Those who gathered for the meeting at the Barcelona restaurant on 11 April included Buckland-Wright, Agar, Banting, Baxter, Brunius, Hayter, Howard, McWilliam, Onslow-Ford, Sewter, Colquhoun, Jennings, Lye, Mesens, Nash, Read, Penrose, and Remington. Half of the people who attended had agreed to exhibit at the abortive Stafford Gallery exhibition. Despite McWilliam's refusal to exhibit, he attended the dinner. On the other hand, although Cecil Collins had agreed to exhibit, he could not attend the dinner, but wanted to know what had been said during the meeting. The discussion focused on the position of Surrealists' position in, and towards, the art world and determined that the artist should be allowed to exhibit his work wherever possible, the British Art Centre being one of the possible venues. This was strongly supported by Agar and Colquhoun.

Ultimately, the aim of the Barcelona meeting was to try and refocus Surrealist activity. As Remy stated in *Surrealism in Britain in the thirties: angels of anarchy and machines for making clouds*, "Not only was it a way of seeing 'who was for and who was against', but it was also an attempt to define a policy which would guarantee and protect the group's intransigence in the chaos of wartime." The idea behind this meeting was "that, in the ideological and material confusion prevailing in the first months of war, Surrealists should define their stance both as individuals and as a group."

Mesens had not been invited to participate in the Stafford Gallery exhibition because the couple knew that he would have seen the British Art Centre as a rival to the London Gallery and disapproved of their association with Guggenheim. He had been scathing about the motives for founding the British Art Centre in 1939. But he attended the Barcelona meeting and took the opportunity to declare that "one cannot reproach anyone for covering himself materially, that is to say for undertaking certain work without special significance but satisfying his immediate necessities," yet "some of us have gone beyond." Clearly, this was a jibe at Pailthorpe and Mednikoff, from whom he was determined to distance himself. He went on:

> I assert that all flirting with the art world is the most crucial outrage against all the perspectives the surrealist movement has had in view since its advent [...] In order to give all the force necessary to a surrealist activity, are you prepared to renounce all participation in group exhibitions springing from an artistic bourgeois spirit? Are you prepared to withdraw your name from the membership list of organisations offering the kind of the AIA, the London Group, the British Art Centre.

He thus made his hostility to Guggenheim and anything involving her crystal clear.

Confronted by the challenge to his authority as the leader of the British Surrealists through Mednikoff's and Pailthorpe's scheme, Mesens mounted a counterattack at the Barcelona meeting and demanded allegiance to a number of propositions. Anyone wishing to remain in the British Surrealist group would have to commit to the following rules:

1 Adherence to the proletarian revolution
2 Agreement not to join any group or association, professional or other, including any secret society, other than the surrealist
3 Agreement not to exhibit or publish except under surrealist auspices.

Pailthorpe, Mednikoff, and Colquhoun objected to the final point because, in effect, it meant not publishing or exhibiting at all now that the London Gallery had closed. *London Bulletin* was at the point of folding.

The day after the meeting at the Barcelona restaurant Colquhoun wrote another letter to Mednikoff:

Dear Mednikoff,

I hope you will let me know any developments that may arise from last night's meeting. At the finish the result was by no means clear.

My impression was that the main split was not due to differences on political theory and practice, but to divergence of view as to how Surrealism should approach the public. The view of yourself and Dr Pailthorpe is, I gather, that we should put Surrealism before the public as much as possible, exhibit, no matter neither where nor with whom. Mesens counters this with trying to prevent us exhibiting in any shows, or contributing to any reviews, without his blessing.

As regards politics, I don't think the issue is pressing - there are some members who like to mention Revolution and the Proletariat sometimes; but no one has either the desire or the ability for effective political action. Everyone is, however, agreed in a basic revolutionary feeling.

As for the two views on how to give one's work to the public, most members are between the two extremes, some near to you, some to Mesens. I myself feel that Mesens cannot attempt to limit our field of activity unless he can offer some alternative. What we need is a review, and a permanent gallery which continually shows surrealist work. It would also be very useful, for those interested in the scientific side, to meet for research and discussion.

I think the first essential is for a group to be formed, and even this was not finally decided upon; next we could discuss how to act. I myself think Penrose's suggestion of an exhibition in Zwemmer's a good one; I feel, and have always felt, rather doubtful about any exhibiting at the B.A.C, which entails membership of that organization, but I am not definite by deciding against it. I think we might consider exhibiting in mixed shows, such as the recent one at Burlington House, but as a group, having a room or wall to ourselves and one or more of our members to hang our pictures and act for us on the committee. In this way a protest could be made without dissipating our efforts.

I hope what I've said may be of use. Do let me know when you and Dr Pailthorpe are next in London, and we could meet. Hoping that some definite results may be attained.

Yours sincerely
Ithell Colquhoun

The letter demonstrates the two major factions within the group due to a 'divergence of view as to how Surrealism should approach the public' with Pailthorpe, Mednikoff, Agar, and Colquhoun wanting to "exhibit, no matter neither where nor with whom" and with Mesens trying to prevent members from 'exhibiting in any shows, or contributing to any reviews, without his blessing'. Penrose's counter-suggestion for an exhibition to be mounted at the Zwemmer Gallery implies that he was between the two extremes.

Penrose favoured Anton Zwemmer's gallery because, together with Mesens and Peter Watson, he was the co-director of the gallery and, at the time, it was credited as one of the galleries that had done the most to introduce Surrealism to England. Moreover, Zwemmer and Penrose had also bought the London Gallery in April 1938. Indeed, in a tribute to Zwemmer on his 70th birthday, Penrose stated how he saw Zwemmer as the person who, in the 1930s, when Surrealism was belatedly coming to London 'made it possible for our small group of poets and artists to exhibit our works and publish our manifestos at a time when no one else had the courage or the foresight to do so.'

Clearly, the Barcelona meeting resulted in loyalties being severely tested as many individual members of the Surrealist movement continued to correspond and meet privately. A letter from Colquhoun to Mednikoff, dated 3 May, refers to these more private meetings: "Have you heard any more details about what happened at the 'secret' meeting; and have any more been held since? I have tried to find out, but have heard nothing from anyone." Another letter, dated 8 May, from Read, who was himself to be excluded by Mesens from the Surrealist group at a date still to be established, again alludes to these secret meetings. The letter also informs us that even after Mesens's demand for Surrealists to exhibit only under the auspices of the Surrealist group, Pailthorpe and Mednikoff were still keen on organising the Stafford Gallery exhibition:

Dear Mr. Mednikoff,

I did not hear very much about the secret session - Sewter was very discreet, and Penrose, whom I have seen since, very conciliatory. I shall see Moore tomorrow, and I gather he is all for avoiding an open breach in the movement. Mesens is the only disturber of the peace, though he easily influences Penrose. I am glad you are going ahead with the exhibition - I think it is the only thing to do, and you are doing it on the right line.

These letters reveal that several 'secret sessions' were being held at the time and, due to Pailthorpe and Mednikoff's refusal to agree to Mesens's terms, it is likely that these private meetings were where the future of the couple's involvement with the Surrealist group was sealed. Read's letter also reflects the dynamics of his relationship with the couple. As an anarchist, he would not have been troubled by their lack of political alignment, and the letters which they exchanged show that Read believed that their scientific work was truly revolutionary in its own way.

Ironically, despite all the drama it had caused, the proposed exhibition was never held, as Story closed the Stafford Gallery on 8 June 1940. An undated letter to Mednikoff from Story confirms that the Executive Committee decided to close the British Art Centre for the Summer months and to re-open in Autumn. The reason she gave was that the Committee had organised an exhibition of contemporary British paintings and it was being taken to the USA. Story claimed that the gallery hoped that the results of showing the artists' work in America would mean an extended market and greater appreciation for British painting in the United States. No doubt, the war lay behind her decision to exhibit British works in America instead of London, where it had become virtually impossible to maintain the art market.

Mesens's hard-line position precipitated a general drift away from the group, headed by Pailthorpe, Mednikoff, and Colquhoun. Read, who had been more drawn to anarchism than to Surrealism for some time, was equally unprepared to comply with the third condition Mesens stipulated but remained loosely affiliate. Due to their objections to Mesens's demands, Read, Colquhoun, Pailthorpe, and Mednikoff were not invited to participate in the 'Surrealism Today' exhibition at the Zwemmer Gallery, which was held from 13 June to 3 July 1940. By agreeing to organise and participate in this exhibition, Penrose showed that he supported Mesens's decisions and was not willing to ask the couple to exhibit. The redefined outlook of the Surrealist movement was also emphasised in the final issue of the *London Bulletin*, which coincided with the exhibition. It was published under the directorship of Mesens, Penrose, and Onslow-Ford, with Penrose financing most of it. Together with Agar, he had also designed the window display of the Zwemmer Gallery. Clearly, Penrose was still determined to further the activities of the Surrealist group. The triple issue included texts by Melville, Onslow-Ford, and Maddox, poems by Péret and Eluard, and pieces by Breton, Mesens, and Mabille. The cover page reads:

Fight Hitler and his ideology wherever it appears. You must.
His defeat is the indispensable prelude to the total liberation
    of humanity.

Read's letter to Mednikoff on 8 May, 1940 also confirms that, during that period, Pailthorpe was focusing on publishing her work and that plans for her to publish her book, 'The Geography of Phantasy,' in America were already being suggested. He wrote:

I read the Synopsis with great interest and have now passed it on to the other directors of Routledge. But the publishing situation is now extremely difficult. We are reduced to 15% of last year's paper consumption, and there is talk of a further reduction and even a censorship of books. Meanwhile costs are going up. If the situation continues for any length of time, English literature will have to move bodily to America, and I think your best plan is to begin at that end. I don't know what Dr Pailthorpe's contacts are there, but I seem to remember that she said she did contemplate the necessity of going over to arrange for American publication.

Herbert Read

Read's involvement in the publication of Pailthorpe's book confirms his genuine interest in her work, and as a co-director of Routledge, it was natural that she appealed to him for his help. In another letter, Read goes on to say:

Dear Dr Pailthorpe,

I have had a further discussion with the Directors [of Routledge] about 'The Geography of Phantasy'. They suggest that the best plan would be for you to prepare a synopsis or description of a preliminary volume, stating the minimum number of words and of illustrations which you require. We would then write to Norton and see if we can come to some arrangement with them for joint publication.

I think you will agree that this is the better plan.

With kind regards,

Yours sincerely,

Herbert Read

Pailthorpe's reply to Read was:

Dear Mr. Read,

I am enclosing a descriptive synopsis of the book, as requested, for submitting to Mr. Norton (American Publisher).

I am also sending you a sort of 'blurb' about the origin of the research, adding an outline of my career and an abstract from the world-wide press publicity that my previous book brought me - all to be used at your discretion. I am still getting press notices from time to time.

Should Mr. Norton not wish to co-operate with you will you kindly get him to return the synopsis.

In the meantime I sincerely hope he will come to an agreement about publication.

Kindest regards,

Yours very sincerely

Although 'The Geography of Phantasy' evidently dealt with her psycho-analytic research, there is no trace of the manuscript. For this reason, it is not known whether the book had been completed or whether Pailthorpe only went so far as to draft a synopsis. There is also no evidence that any of the documents she refers to in the letter above still survive. Although 'The Geography of Phantasy' was not published, their correspondence demonstrates that Read played an important role in helping her publish her work. In addition, Read was also involved in the couple's move to New York. In a letter to the publisher Frank Norton, he wrote:

Dear Frank,

This is to introduce to you Dr Pailthorpe, a good friend of a very distinguished psychologist and mine. She is coming to New York to arrange the publication of a book dealing with her psychoanalytical researches, which are of a fundamental and perhaps revolutionary character. She has introductions to one or two other publishers, but you too may be interested, and in any case you would be interested to meet Dr Pailthorpe. Routledge is interested in the British rights, but that we can discuss later if necessary.

I wrote to you the other day, but this note may reach you earlier. So this is an opportunity to reassure you that we are all still well and not too overwhelmed by events.

Yours ever

Herbert Read

Other letters written at the time show that Pailthorpe was making plans to move to America. Several factors prompted their desire to move to America. In 1940 there was an exodus to America because it was seen as a safe English-speaking haven with an interest in Surrealism. Opportunities had dried up in England because of the war, and many Surrealists were going to America instead. The couple's disenchantment with Surrealism in Britain and Pailthorpe's desire to publish her book also contributed to their move. In a letter to an unknown organisation, dated 29 June 1940, E.T. Jensen, the Chairman of the Institute for the Scientific Treatment of Delinquency, wrote that Pailthorpe asked for a permit to leave the country with Mednikoff. He wrote that she was engaged in the final stages of work in relation to new and profound medical research and that the William C. Whitney Foundation in New York had invited the couple to complete the undertaking in America. The William C. Whitney Foundation was set up in 1937 by Dorothy Whitney, the daughter of the American businessman and statesman William Whitney. One of the wealthiest women in America at the time, she was a benefactor of the arts and of feminist and pacifist causes, and a supporter of social and labour reform. She also lent financial support to progressive alternative education and scholarly research. The Foundation still exists today and consists of works collected by Dorothy and her husband Leonard Elmhirst. They were believed to be the most substantial private patrons of architecture, the arts, and education in the twentieth century in England.

Although it is not known who recommended the couple to the Foundation, in his letter E.T. Jensen stated:

> The Foundation are supplying the necessary affidavit pledging their complete support for the period of one year.
>
> It is essential not only that the research material be put out of reach of destruction, but also that both Dr Pailthorpe and Mr. Mednikoff be safeguarded as they alone could apply the new technique of treatment, which is the outcome of the research, and prepare the research material for presentation to the medical world, an important task which remains to be accomplished.
>
> It is recognised that the most advanced knowledge in psychology must be basic to the understanding of social, political and economic problems. I believe that this work is so outstanding as to be of national importance and indeed to be valuable for a higher type of propaganda.

Moreover, a letter from Anna Bogue, the secretary of the William C. Whitney Foundation, to Pailthorpe on 25 October 1940 states that the Foundation had allocated a $2000 grant to enable the couple to move to America and explore the possibilities of organising their material and publishing her book. Another letter to an unknown addressee from the President of the Medical Society of Individual Psychology, Sir Walter Langdon-Brown, also confirms that some publishers were interested in Pailthorpe's work.

On 17 July 1940, Sir Frederick Whyte, the Director of the American Division of the Ministry of Information in London, wrote a letter to an unidentified source:

> This is to certify that the bearer of this letter, Dr Pailthorpe, and her assistant Mr. Mednikoff, are visiting the United States of America for the purposes of medical research work and the preparation of a book for publication. The Ministry of Information has received evidence as to the scientific importance of this work and is anxious that every legitimate assistance should be given to Dr Pailthorpe and Mr. Mednikoff.

In a second letter, also dated 17 July 1940, Whyte asked if Pailthorpe's papers, drawings, and paintings could be quickly passed for export to the United States on the grounds that they "are of scientific value only, and are essential to the important medical research which Dr Pailthorpe and her assistant, Mr. Mednikoff, are carrying on, for the purpose of which they have been given permission to visit the United States." The use of the word 'assistant' in both letters insinuates that Pailthorpe assumed the position of the driving motor when focusing on the scientific aspect of Surrealism. Whereas before the couple's relationship was one of equals, the word 'assistant' implies that Pailthorpe was taking the leading role at that point.

Apart from Whyte's letter, another letter dated 21 October 1940, clarifies that the secretary of the British Institute of Psychoanalysis, Sylvia Payne, had also encouraged Pailthorpe to move to the United States and publish her research so that others could have the opportunity to consider her technique in "the study of the unconscious origin of artistic impulses." A telegram, reflecting the continuing closeness of Pailthorpe and Dimsdale, also confirms that in 1940 Dimsdale sent Pailthorpe £500 to New York to fund her research costs there. There is no record of the couple having any further contact with Read following their move to New York or mention of the publication of 'The Geography of Phantasy.'

Clearly, although the meeting at the Barcelona restaurant resulted in purges and ideological splits within the English movement as well as the departure of Colquhoun, Mednikoff, and Pailthorpe, it also meant a revitalisation of the group, as was demonstrated by the Zwemmer Gallery exhibition of June 1940. Evidently, as Louisa Buck said, "In its demands for an unblinking commitment, the British Surrealist Group could not accommodate many of these determined individuals who were taking their own form of Surrealism in directions that were unconventional and challenging." Because of this, the couple's commitment to the pursuit of science in their psychoanalytical experiments was deemed intolerable.

The couple's refusal to exhibit and publish only with the backing of the Surrealist group following Mesens's demands at the Barcelona meeting on 11 April 1940, resulted in them never being connected to the British group again. Although Anthony Penrose and Nigel Walsh have claimed that they were expelled from the group, no record of such an expulsion has come to light. Nor are there records of who may have encouraged the expulsion or supported the couple. They may have left of their own accord. Expelled or not, they left England for New York on 24 July 1940 and were never again associated with the Surrealist group. After their departure, Pailthorpe and Mednikoff kept to their vow not to join any other group or organisation for the rest of their lives, which they spent in close collaboration.

The Fall of France in June 1940 had inevitably led to further disruption of the Surrealist group headed by Breton. The slide in Britain was more pronounced in France because of the Occupation and caused difficulty in maintaining group ethos and action. Because of their involvement in what the Nazis had condemned as 'degenerate' art, as well as their affiliation with Communism, the Surrealists in France were in a particularly vulnerable position and a number of them, including Breton, Duchamp, Mabille, Masson, and Dominguez, made their way to Marseille in an attempt to reach the United States. Two months later, on 21 August, Stalin's agents assassinated Trotsky in Mexico. Penrose stayed in London throughout the war, and his home in Downshire Hill was frequented by many Surrealist friends from France. He first served as an air-raid warden on night duty in Hampstead and then as a war office instructor in camouflage to the Home Guard.

The political arguments, alliances, and biases within the British and French Surrealist groups make up a complex history. Political solidarity was short-lived as the alignment shifted among the various factions. The main conflicts centred on the attitude Surrealists should take towards the Communist party, as well as the growing divisive demands of Mesens in England and Breton in France. Hence, there could never be any hope of agreement. These conflicts led to internal tension and hostility within both groups and resulted in various alliances being formed. The dogmatic views of Mesens and Breton allowed no compromise. Splits, expulsions, and defections occurred while the decision of leading figures, including Breton, to choose exile in North America inevitably made the pursuit of group activity extremely difficult, if not impossible.

Note

1 A different English translation by Dwight MacDonald was also published in *Partisan Review,* New York, IV, no. 1, Fall 1938: 49–53. The *London Bulletin* translation was not the one that Henderson translated but another version. It does not state who translated the text.

11   The couple's move to North America

The measure adopted by the English government during the Second World War caused interruptions and delays that greatly hindered Pailthorpe's research work at a "moment when uninterrupted work was vital to [its] progress (...), and these breaks in continuity often spoil several months work" (Pailthorpe, Letter dated December 28, 1942). So, under "the urgency of procuring both the completion of the research and the safety of the material, which is quite irreplaceable," Pailthorpe and Mednikoff (who volunteered for army service but was rejected as being medically unfit) moved away from the risk of destruction through bombing "to the safety of the United States" (ibid.) on July 20 1940, sailing from Liverpool Harbour to New York.

Pailthorpe and Mednikoff moved to the United States with the blessing of the British Government and the medical profession since their research was felt to be of great importance as demonstrated by three letters of support from Walter Langdon-Brown (Regius Professor of Physics at the University of Cambridge) (see Box 11.1), Lord Thomas Jeeves Horder (president of the British Eugenics Society and of the Cremation Society of Great Britain; he was the personal physician of three prime ministers of the United Kingdom) (see Box 11.2), and Ernest Thomas Jensen (founder and honorary secretary of the Tropical Diseases Prevention Association, Fellow of the Society of Tropical Medicine and Hygiene, and co-founder, Vice-President and Chairman of the Executive Council of the ISTD) (see Box 11.3).

After an initial period spent in the Big Apple where they showed some of their works at the first exhibition of British, Canadian, and American Contemporary Art held at the American Art Centre in January–February 1941, Pailthorpe and Mednikoff moved to Berkeley in Northern California. During their time there, the couple continued their research on the therapeutic aspect of art as they were granted a loan from the William C. Whitney Foundation for the period dating from December 1940 to September 1942. In Northern California Pailthorpe was a frequent visitor to both Berkeley and San Francisco University libraries for research purposes. In the Summer of 1942, following the advice of Peggy Guggenheim, Pailthorpe and Mednikoff spent their holidays in British Columbia where, because of their fascination with the

DOI: 10.4324/9781003427032-12

Box 11.1

July 1, 1940

I desire strongly to support Dr. G.W. Pailthorpe's application for permission to leave this country in order to go to the United States to carry on research work of a highly specialised kind on psychological lines.

Owing to the difficulties in carrying on the publication of this work in Great Britain during the war, she is trying to arrange to get over to the United States where two or three publishers are already interested in her research.

You will find from her professional record in the Medical Directory that she is highly qualified to carry on work of this kind and has been a research worker under the Medical Research Council.

I have been more particularly interested in her work on the scientific investigation of delinquency and many may remember that her book entitled "What We Put In Prison" published in 1932 created a great deal of interest and played an important part in leading to some humanitarian reforms.

I should like to emphasise the importance of her work which has received such recognition in responsible quarters. I have read Dr. Jensen's letter addressed to the Home Secretary and am in agreement with what he states therein as to her work and its significance particularly at the present juncture. I therefore hope it may be possible for her to receive support in furtherance thereof.

Signed: W. Langdon-Brown,
M.D. D.Sc., F.R.C.P.

Box 11.2

July 8, 1940.

I am desirous of supporting Dr. Grace Pailthorpe's application for a permit to go to America with the object of publishing the results of her recent research into the psychology of the present conditions in respect of children here and in the other parts of Europe.

I regard such work as being of National importance and the sooner the results are in our hands the better.

Signed: Horder, M.D., F.R.C.P., etc.

Box 11.3

July 20, 1940.

Dr. Grace W. Pailthorpe, whose reputation is world-wide, conducted research on inmates of Holloway Prison for the Medical Research Council under the auspices of the Home Office. Her report was published by H.M Stationery Office.

Her book 'What We Put In Prison' attracted notice in many countries. It was my privilege to be associated with her then in regard to these publications and immediately afterwards in the foundation of the Institute for Scientific Treatment of Delinquency which now, ten years later, has achieved a powerful and honourable position in the esteem of government, legal and medical professions as well as the public.

Besides its recognised function in assisting the Courts, treating delinquents, and conducting research, it has become an authorised teaching body for the instruction of doctors and laymen working for the Courts and dependent organisations. Its seed is germinating here and in distant lands.

Subsequently Dr. Pailthorpe has been engaged in research of such importance as to result in the elaboration of a new system of psychology which may be considered epoch-making, in that its application alters the subject's whole social outlook and enables him to understand how all the working of mind-function occurs from the infant-stage onwards.

It is recognised that the most advanced knowledge in psychology is basic to understanding of all social, political and economic problems.

The findings of this research are so outstanding as to be of national importance and, indeed at present to be valuable for a higher type of propaganda. They must appeal to a rapidly increasing number of intellectuals who, with the material, may pave the way to universal peace. This work will be acclaimed by all who strive and pray for this ideal and my sincerest wish is that they may accord active support in the endeavour of attainment.

Signed: F. T. Jensen,
M.B. (Lond.) M.R.C.S., L.R.C.P.
Chairman of Council
Institute for the Scientific
Treatment of Delinquency.

Rocky Mountains and since the region was the nearest to England on that side of the Atlantic, they then decided to settle there at the end of September (Zemans, 1981).

Pailthorpe and Mednikoff were both given six-month permits to leave the United States. However, when they were leaving, Mednikoff was stopped at the border in Blain (Washington) and was informed that he had to also have permission from his local Selective Service Board to leave. The immigration official advised Mednikoff to contact the place where he had registered, which was in New York. A few days later, Mednikoff received a telephone call at his hotel from the Immigration Office on the border and was told that such permission had been granted. He was allowed to go to Canada, but no written permission was given to him.

Once they moved to Vancouver, Pailthorpe immediately found a job at the provincial psychiatric hospital (later Riverview Hospital)—which at the time was acknowledged as a model of psychiatric health care—where she worked until April 1943 (Walsh & Wilson, 1998). The facility hosted a few thousand patients and consisted of, among other units, the Boys' Industrial School for juvenile delinquents and the Acute Psychopathic Unit. The hospital was located in Essondale (one of Vancouver's suburbs) where Pailthorpe commuted via public transportation on a daily basis. She was the only female doctor in the hospital and was recognised as one of the leading psychiatrists and alienists. Mednikoff too worked at the hospital as her technical assistant.

As the date for a renewal of Mednikoff's permit approached, Pailthorpe wrote to the New York Selective Service Board asking for a permanent deferment for an indefinite period for Mednikoff. She requested that they let her know to whom she should refer if they could not grant it. Having had no reply to that question and having a recollection of having heard that it was allowable to refer to the President of the United States for a matter of that kind, Pailthorpe eventually did so at the end of January 1943. In several letters, Pailthorpe described Mednikoff as "a key man in this research" and stated that "without him the research cannot be completed" (e.g., Letter to the President of the United States, dated January 31st, 1943 [Pailthorpe, 1942–1943]). It is unclear whether it was this letter which allowed the procedure to progress, but in February of that year Mednikoff was granted permanent residency, bringing an end to a situation that could have jeopardised their research and its positive completion.

In 1943 while in British Columbia, Pailthorpe founded the Association for the Scientific Treatment of Delinquency (ASTD), whose objectives over-lapped those of the ISTD in London. Its specific focus was juvenile delinquency. Indeed, an objective of the ASTD was to provide assistance to the courts and, most importantly, to parents who wanted immediate help for their delinquent children as it would avoid even worse consequences. As president of the ASTD, Pailthorpe held various lectures (for example, "Delinquency begins in the cradle" and "Causes and prevention of crime"), and spoke at conferences (for example, on "Penal reform") and round-tables (for example at the 1944 annual meeting of the John Howard Society on "What about our criminals?"). As seen below, Boxes 11.4 and 11.5 include two papers titled, respectively, "Delinquency is curable" (originally intended for publication in the News Herald) and "the Association for the Scientific Treatment of Delinquency presents an argument and plan for demobilising

Box 11.4

Delinquency is curable

Some time ago, in the columns of a Vancouver newspaper, the mother of a wayward son publicly charged the community with part of the guilt for her son's delinquency. She was entirely justified.

She said also, "There should be some place where a mother can go when she feels that her son or daughter is heading for trouble ..." "If there were only some type of establishment where parents could place their children for proper guidance and supervision when faced with problems like this ... where they could receive essential training in the right direction without the embarrassment or shame of publicly punitive measure." Much more was said, but the most important points are in these quoted remarks, with which I fully agree.

This mother – and many others too, no doubt, – will be glad to know that not very long ago an Association for the Scientific Treatment of Delinquency (ASTD.) was formed in Vancouver with just those very aims in view, namely, to provide a place for delinquent children and young adults to be brought for treatment. This public-spirited body of people realises fully that parents need help in such matters.

Much is already known by psychologically trained doctors about the way the mind functions – why a child who has usually behaved well should suddenly become a 'problem.' Such doctors can, by understanding questioning and treatment of a delinquent, discover the causes of his or her behaviour, and, by means of re-education, help the erring youngster to conform to social standards.

It is the aim of the ASTD to get the public to realise this; and to demand that the city of Vancouver plan such an establishment and staff it with properly trained personnel.

You will probably ask, how would an organisation of this kind function? To answer this let me tell you of the Institute for the Scientific Treatment of Delinquency (ISTD) in London, England, which is the example we in Vancouver are trying to follow.

The ISTD was formed by doctors trained in psychotherapy. They gave their services without thought of monetary gain. After six years of persistent endeavour they became known throughout the world as a group of workers who successfully cure delinquents of their anti-social behaviour. Free psychotherapeutic treatment was given to those brought to them by parents seeking advice and help. They likewise treated youthful and adult offenders sent by magistrates, probation officers and school teachers. Series of lectures also were given to magistrates, probation officers, lawyers, and so on. Educating the servants of the public, as well as the public, to an understanding of the true facts underlying criminal behaviour was an integral part of the programme of the ISTD.

Now a word about the personnel. Both psychotherapists and psychiatrists are needed in an institution of this kind: but chiefly the need is for psychotherapists (medical and authorised lay psychotherapists), for these trained people are the ones who do most of the treatment. A psychotherapist is not necessarily a psychiatrist, nor is a psychiatrist a psychotherapist. Psychiatry and psychology are two separate approaches to the same branch of learning.

The psychotherapist approaches his patients as one whose mental behaviour has been warped by some early childhood incidents or conditions. He searches for links that will lead to the early childhood experiences that started the 'rot.' When he gets there, he helps the patient to understand how he has been reacting to his early experiences. With understanding the behaviour, the delinquent becomes non-delinquent. He is cured of the criminal tendencies that got him into trouble.

A physical examination is first given to each patient brought to the Institution. If no physical signs are present to explain the anti-social behaviour the patient is passed on to the psychotherapist. There are usually psychotherapists of every school of psychology at hand to help such patients. Working with these doctors are social workers who search out the background to every case – the financial condition of the family, the kind of house, surroundings and district the family live in, and so on. Every angle of the case is carefully gone into, collected and recorded. The social worker saves the doctors a great deal of time by gathering this information in advance.

As the greatest number of delinquents have been found to need psychotherapeutic treatment it is obvious that such trained people should be encouraged to come to Vancouver since there is a great need for them.

To the parents of Vancouver, I offer this as a solution to your delinquency problem. Get your psychotherapists, psychiatrists and social workers banded together as a team, and then make it financially possible for them to do the work. When such a group is fully organised and in action, the various clubs and recreational centres in this city will be called upon to do their part.

The ASTD is working hard to get the public interested enough to support this project. Only when proper support is forthcoming will it be possible to start a clinic where delinquent children and adults can be treated by fully trained psychotherapists.

So to all of you who deplore the appalling amount of delinquency in this city, I offer this advice: act now by giving your support to this Assoc.'s efforts to educate the public to this need, your donation to help pay the expenses of this work. Membership to the Assoc. is also invited.

(Pailthorpe, 1942–44)

Box 11.5

The Association for the Scientific Treatment of Delinquency presents an argument and plan for demobilising criminals

The argument

When a Chief Justice of the Province, speaking to a man he is sentencing, says, "To my mind it is a pity medical science has not so far advanced as to treat this quirk in your mind (criminal behaviour of a confirmed character) so you could be of use to the country instead of disgrace," it is unfair to blame the ordinary man and woman for ignorance of the fact that medical science has already for more than a generation been curing people of such tendencies, when our judiciary authorities are so uninformed.

The above statement by the Chief Justice emphasises the imperative need for instructing all judiciary officials, law-makers, and law-enforcers of the existence of scientific methods for the cure and prevention of crime.

It is equally imperative a need to inform you, the general public, of the fact that not only can criminal tendencies be prevented, when treated early enough, but that established anti-social behaviour can be cured ... and that it is cheaper and more effective to cure the criminal than to imprison him and then release him when his compulsion to do damage has been augmented by hate due to the irrational punishment inflicted on him.

It is cheaper to spend money in curing the criminal once and for all than to spend money in imprisoning a person many times.

Imprisonment is a waste of money for it does not prevent a criminal repeating an offence. For example, a 63-year-old woman who recently was released on parole after 18 years of imprisonment for murdering a man, immediately murdered the woman to whom she had been paroled.

In Vancouver last year a magistrate said to the prisoner he was sentencing, "You are very expensive luxury to the taxpayers. As I look over your record I find that there have been a total of 86 convictions laid against you."

It has been shown that the average cost of repeaters of crime to the State is 25,000 dollars per head (vide Report of the Royal Commission to Investigate the Penal System of Canada, 1938).

Apart from the damage and useless expenditure of your money there is also the preventable misery that individuals and families suffer when a crime is committed by one of its members.

Think of the needless misery we force our children to suffer! Only unhappy children give trouble. The children that are dragged to our Juvenile Courts to be 'punished' for some anti-social acts are always unhappy mortals expressing their disapproval of being frustrated or uncared for.

It is not enough to say the child has poor parents, or that he or she is not loved by them, or is influenced by bad friends and surroundings, or is an orphan, or has an inferiority complex, and then still treat the child as a criminal. It is time delinquent children be treated medically and psychologically; and, where parents are also at fault, ignorantly or otherwise, that they be given proper advice and *assistance* in relation to the child's future. *Advice without treatment* is as useless as imprisonment without cure.

The plan

Medical and psychological knowledge has taught us that criminals are curable, and that the majority are psychologically maladjusted. So long as we allow our treatment of criminals to continue in the mediaeval way we do today, we are ourselves guilty of criminal neglect. What then are we going to do about it? What can we do about it?

We need: –

OBSERVATION CENTRES and CLINICS properly equipped and staffed for the diagnosis and treatment of delinquents.

To provide TRAINING FACILITIES for students in the scientific study of delinquency and crime.

Psychologists and psychiatrists to ASSIST THE COURTS and GOVERNMENT DEPARTMENTS by the preliminary investigation of the physical and mental condition of each convicted person, and a statement from them of the TREATMENT REQUIRED.

To provide PAMPHLETS, LECTURES, and DISCUSSIONS to educate public opinion on delinquency and its prevention and cure.

Such OBSERVATION CENTRES and CLINICS would prevent future cases such as the following occurring: –

"Police today filed seven charges of murder against Charles Bohme, 44-year-old crippled factory worker, who confessed to setting 27 fires since July 15 1955."

Seven murders because of a psychological compulsion to start fires. Charles could have been sent to such a Clinic when he was a child. Parents usually know when their children's behaviour is peculiar or 'difficult.' But we must provide the Observation Centre and Clinic, otherwise parents and guardians are helpless.

Last of all there are the veterans of this war who, conditioned to acts of violence, will be among our future criminals. Are we going to condemn to prison those who we have so laboriously made into criminals in order that they should save our lives? Dare we treat them so scurrilously when we know that psychological treatment will help them?

Will you help us make an Observation Centre and Clinic possible? Your immediate donations and co-operation will assist us in spreading the knowledge that science has provided the tools with which to eradicate this social evil – preventable crime. Your immediate donations and co-operation will help us build up a public demand for radical change in the treatment of social misfits.

Your donations and membership are urgently needed. Won't you fill in the attached form (overleaf) immediately and mail it to our treasurer? Help us in our plan to make your children and your future secure … secure from preventable crime.

(Pailthorpe, 1942–44)

criminals," in which Pailthorpe outlines the background, aims, and functioning of the ASTD.

The 'automatic' artistic therapy which characterised the clinical approach of the ASTD drew the attention of the Ladies' Auxiliary of the Vancouver Art Gallery (the largest museum in Western Canada) who, in 1944, invited Pailthorpe to talk about Surrealism. What is still not certain is whether a painter of such standing as Pailthorpe had to some extent already integrated within Vancouver's artistic milieu; though evidence shows that this group of volunteer workers and art-lovers from Essondale were the first to invite her, approximately two years after her move there, to talk about her work (Larocque, 2007).

In her first public talk, dated 14 April 1944, Pailthorpe's (1944a) lecture (the first lecture ever given at the VAG by a surrealist artist), which was followed by a slideshow and a public discussion, provided the Western Canadian mass media with a first definition, albeit concise, of Surrealist Art as the expression of the subconscious. Pailthorpe's explanation of Surrealist Art emphasised its purely psychic and automatic nature as well as its means of expressing the real process of thought. Morovere, she predicted that "in the future this type of art will come into the education of the young" (Vancouver Sun, April 15, 1944, p. 3), adding that it is easier for the child to express himself, than for an adult who has already created a prison wall around his unconscious fears. She also said that "If we can keep open the unconscious for the growing child we are going to keep open all that creative urge everyone feels but few are able to enjoy" (ibid.). The event sold out and several people were turned away (for the second time in the gallery's history).

A second talk, dated 13 June 1944, took place at the inauguration of Pailthorpe's and Mednikoff's joint exhibition of their works (June 13–July 2 1944). The content matched those of her first lecture. Here, she stated: "it is of the utmost importance that the 'unconscious' or hidden, repressed part of our minds, should find release and expression" (News Herald, June 14, 1944), adding that the "unconscious (…) never repeats itself" (Vancouver Sun, June 14, 1944, p. 13). This viewpoint is what she had previously discussed in depth (Pailthorpe, 1938–39). It was the first Surrealist exhibition held in this part of the Rocky Mountains. It consisted of about 80 works, most of which were in black-and-white, and some in colour (described by the press as having "a special fascination"; Vancouver Sun, June 14, 1944, p. 13), yet "All give a feeling of sincerity on the part of the artist. Here, the spectator feels, is no striving after effect" (ibid.). Interestingly, all the paintings were kept under glass because, as the Vancouver Sunday Sun (June 10, 1944) reports, when the artists gave their first exhibition in London in 1936, some irritated spectators expressed their anger by writing what they thought of the pictures. However, unlike the very negative reactions showed by spectators during the first exhibition in London and the negative response given by critics six years earlier at the Surrealist exhibition which was held at the Central National Exhibition in Toronto, this time the critics' comments were more favourable. Here, the press wrote: "You can't ignore Surrealism" (Walker, 1944). This was probably also due to both the scientific aspect and the social significance that Pailthorpe conveyed as she asserted that "the use of 'Surrealism' and the unlocking of the unconscious mind can revolutionise, not only the individual, but the whole cultural and educational structure of society" (News Herald, June 14, 1944). Pailthorpe showed no concern or offence by negative criticism. As she said, "It pleases me as well to have my work disliked as liked, for in either case it is a compliment to the work, which is meant to provoke some definite response. After a time, antagonisms subside, and a liking for what had upset you gradually grows" (News Herald, June 14, 1944).

The interest aroused by this exhibition in Vancouver's community was such that the exhibition was extended by a week and the Western branch of the national radio company Canadian Broadcasting Corporation asked Pailthorpe to give a brief (ten-minute) speech on Surrealism for the programme 'Mirror for Women'. Hence, on July 10 1944, Pailthorpe (1944b) introduced her listeners to the history and philosophy of Surrealism and then followed it with a description of the levels of the psyche and their relationship with dreams and irrationality.

Pailthorpe stressed that the unconscious can be represented through automatic writing or drawing. Recalling the method suggested by Breton (1924), she underlined the ease with which such processes can be activated: "Every time you take up a pencil and begin scribbling, while waiting at a telephone for a call and your thoughts are not concentrated on what you are scribbling, you are drawing automatically. You are not consciously aware of what your hand is creating. You are not in a trance, but your mind is not consciously interfering with what your hand is making the pencil do. What you do in that way is automatic and very similar to the way a Surrealist drawing or painting is done" (Pailthorpe, 1944b, p. 93). The resulting scribble is, at the same time, a sort of hieroglyph of the memory and an expression of liberation. Pailthorpe pointed out that these works, which are the fruit of unconscious automatism rather than a conscious fabrication (and therefore mostly of a fictitious nature), are indeed the most significant surrealist art and which, upon first sight, arouse shock and distress in the viewer. Such emotional reactions are due to the unknown nature of what one is faced with, which must be contemplated at length before it can become familiar: "Enjoy it if you can, or, if it repulses you, accept that emotional response (…) go back to the work again and then again." Such a vision of (true) art celebrates "the value of the marvellous and of the beauty of irrational thought and creation" and legitimises the fantasy as "a universal (…) activity that all have a right to enjoy." It also follows that "We are all potential artists, having within us the divine spark that can ignite the creative flame" (Pailthorpe, 1944, p. 94).

Pailthorpe's main contribution to the birth of Canadian Surrealism was that of her favouring the expansion of pictorial automatism within the sphere of English-Canadian media (Zemans, 1981; Larocque, 2007) as well as, indirectly, of the psychoanalytical approach. A lasting impact on artistic practice and, more generally, on the Canadian artistic milieu was later guaranteed by Jock Macdonald's work who, thanks to Pailthorpe's—his lifelong mentor and confidante—help, was able to separate painting from figurativism (Larocque, 2007), becoming freer and more open as well as experiencing a joy in painting hitherto unknown to him (Zemans, 2016).

On June 20 1945, Pailthorpe gave a talk entitled 'Psychological problems of rehabilitation- getting the family together again' in a conference organised by the Parents' Institute at the University of British Columbia. It was part of a series of lectures for parents by child psychologists. Her focus was on soldiers who returned home with psychological problems. In her talk, she stated that soldiers are "told to kill, given the means to kill, and taught every known trick in the art of attacking an opponent." She insisted that it would be a worse crime to imprison those "we have made into criminals in order that they should save our lives." She stressed the need for community centres because she believed that "Creative work is the best treatment for those physically, spiritually and mentally shattered." The following day, a reference to her talk was made in an article entitled 'Army teaches Gangster Arts: Psychiatrist fears crime wave on return of soldiers' and published in the *Vancouver Daily Province* (June 21, 1945).

On November 7 1945, Pailthorpe was asked to participate in a panel meeting (called *Science and Crime*) given by the Vancouver women's school for citizenship and held at Hotel Vancouver. Here, she emphasised the need for a more scientific treatment of delinquency so that eventually prisons would be abolished. She pointed out how this had occurred in England and many prisons were then closed due to a reduction in crime. Her comments on methods of crime punishment were quoted in an article entitled 'Psychologist deplore methods of punishment' and published in *The Vancouver Sun* (November 8, 1945). Another article entitled "Lash is called 'Step Backward' by psycholo-gist" and published in *Vancouver News Herald* (November 8, 1945) emphasised Pailthorpe's assertion that history has shown the "utter uselessness" of the law-makers' approach to solving the problem because, "77 percent of criminals are repeaters" and, "a man is not a criminal until the law makes him so." Both articles referenced her work in England which had led to the closure of prisons.

12 Pailthorpe and Mednikoff's return to England

In March 1946, Pailthorpe and Madnikoff left Vancouver and returned to England where they bought a house in Dorking in Sussex. Mednikoff started working as an antique dealer and Pailthorpe resumed her clinical work as a psychoanalyst. Furthermore, around the first months of 1948, Mednikoff changed his name to Richard Pailthorpe, and the couple began introducing themselves as brother and sister.

Once they returned to England, Pailthorpe withdrew from public life. She remained dedicated to her work as both an artist and as an analyst. Pailthorpe also started doing clinical work as a consultant at the Portman Clinic. She led an art therapy group of 6–8 patients, aged 16–25, from Summer 1948 to December 1952. The group met twice weekly for a three-hour session in the evening. Mednikoff assisted her. From 1950 onwards, Pailthrorpe started referring to herself as a psychologist rather than as a physician. During this period, Pailthorpe and Mednikoff established the first-ever art therapy school in Dorking. In 1951, some of the couple's works were featured in an exhibition at the Artists House Exhibition in London. Other exhibiting artists included Horace Brodzky, Charles Watson, Ronald Dickens, Ateo Casadio, Robin Pitman, and Gwilym Morgan.

Meanwhile "Studies in the Psychology of Delinquency" continued to attract attention. In a letter to Pailthorpe dated 12 September 1951, Professor John W. Tietz from the School of Education at New York University described her work as "a unique and fascinating study." He wrote that her approach to delinquency "opens a new vista of thought" as he had "never seen such a study of the motivational side of delinquency." Unfortunately, no letters written by Pailthorpe in response to Professor Tietz's desire to learn more about her work have surfaced.

During the 1950s, Pailthorpe proved to show much success as an analyst in Sussex. She was called "a distinguished Harley Street Doctor." The fee for six weeks of analysis was £200 (Macdonald, 1954).

Moreover, a letter to Pailthorpe, dated 23 August 1958, from the Hon. Brinsley le Poer Trench shows Pailthorpe's interest in UFO sightings. He was the editor of the *Flying Saucer Review* and he was responding to a letter she had written on 12 August 1958 where she enquired about becoming a member

DOI: 10.4324/9781003427032-13

of the "International UFO Observer Corps." As the chief Investigator of UFO sightings, Brinsley le Poer Trench asked Pailthorpe if she would be willing to take up the post of UFO Area Investigator in Sussex. However, no letter from Pailthorpe in response to this offer has been traced.

13 Pailthorpe's final years

In 1969, almost 20 years after retreating from the artistic scene, Pailthorpe exhibited some of her most recent (produced within the previous three to four years) paintings. This private exhibition was located in the private home of Mr. and Mrs. Gwilym Morgan in Hastings. In an article entitled "She is still a vital artist at 86," published in *Hastings and St Leonard's Observer*, Pailthorpe's paintings were compared to pop art because "they have the same disregard of conventions, the same bold use of colours, the same spontaneity." The writer described her works as having an "invigorating sense of movement" where "each painting is a new discovery" (A62/1/055, June 21, 1969). Another article entitled "Exhibition of recent paintings by Dr. Grace W. Pailthorpe" which was published in *The President's New Bulletin* emphasised the "quality and vitality" as well as the "power and assurance" of her work. The author wrote that "Each painting is an exhilarating adventure in colour, rhythm and fantasy. Dr Pailthorpe's freedom and spontaneity of expression are unusual; her colours and textures are a sheer delight" (Author Unknown, 1969, p. 23).

Two years after this exhibition, Pailthorpe died on July 21, 1971. The cause of her death was cancer. She was 88. In her obituary on Pailthorpe, Helen Sheehan-Dare (a training analyst who supervised, inter alia, Donald Winnicott, Charles Rycroft, and Ignacio Matte Blanco) wrote that Pailthorpe was "the least self-assertive person I have ever met, always more ready to listen than to talk and respecting the opinions of everyone around her. She was far too great an individualist to have ever been completely orthodox in her views, and (…) this independence of thought (…) may (…) have been her most valuable contribution to science" (Sheehan-Dare, 1971, p. 26). An unnamed writer of another obituary published the day after Pailthorpe died stated that her "creative work, painting, was always greatly appreciated by the professional painter who saw in her work the freedom of imagination and technique they themselves wished for. Her painting was always full of richly vital colour." These obituaries show the respect that both Pailthorpe's art and analyst had earned her right until her death.

Soon after Pailthorpe's death, an exhibition called "Britain's Contribution to Surrealism of the 30's and 40's" was held at the Hamet Gallery (3–27 November 1971) in Cork Street, London. It featured works by both

DOI: 10.4324/9781003427032-14

Pailthorpe and Mednikoff. It was the first exhibition to bring together works produced by the majority of the British Surrealists in the 1930s and 1940s. Other exhibiting artists included Eileen Agar, Ithell Colquhoun, Conroy Maddox, ELT Mesens, Henry Moore, Paul Nash, Roland Penrose, and Edith Rimmington. Images of Mednikoff's *Come Back Soon* and Pailthorpe's *The Spotted Ousel* were featured in the exhibition catalogue. The catalogue included a reference to the first International Surrealist Exhibition in London in 1936 and, once again, Breton's admiration of Pailthorpe's works.

Afterword by Glenn Gossling

Grace Pailthorpe was a surgeon in the First World War, an early British psychoanalyst, a ground-breaking criminologist, as well as a surrealist painter, writer, and thinker. Lee Ann Montanaro and Alberto Stefana's *Surrealism and psychoanalysis in Grace Pailthorpe's life and work* is the first detailed biography of Pailthorpe's extraordinary life. Together with their recent companion publication *Grace Pailthorpe's writings on psychoanalysis and Surrealism*, which brings together and makes available a range of her writings, these two volumes represent a significant re-appraisal of an important but near forgotten figure.

A debt of thanks is owed to the National Galleries of Scotland, who have preserved an extensive archive of material on Grace Pailthorpe, and credit has to be given to Lee Ann Montanaro for her almost archaeological efforts to unearth this material on Pailthorpe's life and writings, and bring them to light.

As well as being a talented artist and significant theorist on Surrealism, Pailthorpe was a skilled surgeon, a researcher, an innovative criminologist, and a psychoanalyst. She left a body of artistic work that is now beginning to feature in the collections of major galleries like the Tate and she founded the Portman Clinic,[1] which is internationally recognised for its expertise on forensic psychotherapy, particularly in specialist areas such as violence, delinquency, criminal behaviour, and paraphilias.

The surrealists are perhaps best known as the group of mostly French artists who desired to remake art as a lawless realm modelled on dreams and the unconscious. They drew inspiration from Freud's theories, which at that time were new, controversial and challenged the dominant rationalism of Enlightenment thinking in the way that it de-centred the human subject. André Breton's *Surrealist Manifesto* proposed new ideals that were supposed to redesign the world, free one's mind from the past and from everyday reality to arrive at truths one has never known.

Surrealism sought to actively challenge the restrictive behaviour of societal norms through its imagery, manifestos, and "actions." Sometimes this involved playfully pushing the boundaries, as with Gérard de Nerval taking his pet lobster for a walk on a leash or Salvador Dalí filling a white Rolls Royce with cauliflowers and driving it from Spain to the Sorbonne in Paris to deliver a lecture titled "Phenomenological Aspects of the Paranoiac Critical Method." At other times it involved a more explicitly political engagement such as the surrealist movement's alignment with the Russian revolution arguing that the liberation of humankind and the liberation of the mind could result only from socialist revolution. In this, they are part of a European philosophical tradition that has sought to link social and political emancipation with individual emancipation.

Pailthorpe came to Surrealism not primarily as an artist, but as a doctor and psychoanalytic clinician seeking to improve techniques of diagnosis and treatment; with the belief that "there must be somewhere a quicker way to the deeper layers of the unconscious than by the long drawn-out couch method" (Walsh, 1998). She engaged with the liberatory politics of Surrealism to find a way "to free the psychology of the individual from internal conflict, [and asserted that] the final goal of Surrealism and Psychoanalysis is the same—the liberation of man" (Pailthorpe, 1938–39, p. 53).

It may seem strange that such a pioneering artist, writer, and theorist has all but been forgotten, but her life and work touched on many areas that society would perhaps prefer to remain hidden and buried.

According to Virginia Woolf (1924), "On or about December 1910 human nature changed." The quote is usually associated with the rise of literary modernism and the beginnings of an industrial, technological society, but the period is also significant for psychoanalysis, as Ernest Jones (1910) published the authoritative "Freud's Theory of Dreams" explaining the ideas of Sigmund Freud's *The Interpretation of Dreams* to the English speaking world. This was shortly followed by C. S. Myers' paper on Freud's dream theory to the British Psychological Society in 1912 and the first full translation by A. A. Brill in 1913.[2]

Although nowadays the figure of Freud casts a lengthy shadow over theories of the mind and ideas of unconscious thinking, in Britain at the start of the twentieth century the picture was not so clearly defined. Before the First World War, Freud was just one of many thinkers at the boundaries of philosophy, psychology, and neurology. In fact, at the end of the 19th and start of the twentieth centuries, the thought leaders were very much from France.

In the mid-nineteenth century, French neurologist Jean-Martin Charcot had systematically begun to study hypnosis and hysteria, establishing a famous clinic at Salpêtrière in Paris. Charcot's work was taken forward and developed by a number of his students: Janet, Babinski and ... Freud.

It is from Freud that we have an account of the human mind that came to dominate modern understanding. And for those who studied the mind at that time, Freud was often given "a position no less unique than that which physical science gives to Newton" (Crichton-Miller, 1933).

Freud had studied under Charcot in the mid-1880s and started publishing his own ideas ten years later, coining his own term—psychoanalysis—for the study of the mind and introducing his conception of the unconscious in *The Interpretation of Dreams*, which many consider to be his master-work. However, Freud's ideas were not immediately popular. It took eight years for the original 600 copies of *The Interpretation of Dreams* to sell out (Jenkins, 2017).

His ideas were, if anything, less popular in Britain. In 1911, David Eder, one of the founding members of the Portman Clinic, gave the first-ever psychoanalytic paper to the British Medical Association, and it is said that during his talk on sexual aetiology, the entire medical audience silently walked out so that when he looked up from his notes, he found himself speaking to an empty room.

Psychological medicine and particularly psychoanalysis, with its Mittel-European Jewish roots, were treated with open suspicion if not contempt within the white, Anglo-Saxon, Protestant medical community.

Then came World War 1 (WW1).

A total of 65 million troops from around the world fought in WW1. Eight-and-a-half million troops are thought to have been killed. A total of 21 million troops were wounded. An estimated two million soldiers, sailors, and airmen died from disease, malnutrition, and other causes. An estimated 13 million civilians were killed.

Even now the figures are almost beyond comprehension.

One of the most significant factors in WW1 was the industrialisation of warfare. This kind of warfare had never been seen before and it was shocking. The new weapons and technology that were developed and used led to more death and destruction than any previous war.

Soldiers suffered wounds that were also like nothing doctors had had to deal with before—not only in type, but in scale of numbers. The nature of the injuries forced huge leaps in reconstructive surgery. The very few British surgeons who had specialised in neurology were overwhelmed by the enormous number of head wounds requiring brain surgery (Shepherd, 2000). The war meant that medicine had to catch up to be able to deal with these problems. Among these problems was the impact that the new forms of warfare had on the mind.

By the end of 1914, doctors were finding themselves faced by inexplicable cases: soldiers who were not injured but who had their senses deranged so that they could not see, smell, or taste properly (Shepherd, 2000). Some could not stand or walk, some could not speak and many suffered from the shakes. Between 7 and 10% of officers and 3 to 4% of all ranks were being sent home because of nervous or mental breakdown. No one knew how these symptoms were created (Shepherd, 2000).

Within the British medical profession, there was debate about whether this was caused by physical damage to the nervous system or whether it was emotional shock.

A critical shift occurred when Dr Charles Myers, a distinguished psychologist from Cambridge University, went to France (Shepherd, 2000). Myers, who was a qualified doctor but had never practised, had run the small Cambridge psychology department with William Halse Rivers Rivers and William Mc Dougall (Shepherd, 2000).

Myers had gone to France in 1914 to the hospital at le Touquet in Paris but was frustrated that the other doctors would not let him see any patients (Shepherd, 2000). Because of this, he took the time to visit the French neurologist Dejerine at the Salpêtrière hospital (Shepherd, 2000) and saw a number of cases of soldiers who had been struck dumb or partially paralysed and were made aware of hysterical breakdown (Shepherd, 2000).

Myers returned to le Touquet where, on 5 November 1914, a 20-year-old private soldier was admitted (Myers, 1915). This unknown private became the first recorded case of "shell-shock." Here, Myers was responsible for bringing the term and the condition to the attention of the medical community in his *Lancet* article in 1915 (Kraemer, 2011).

From when the Battle of the Somme took place (July 1916), shell-shock had become a serious drain on manpower, escalating to possibly almost 100,000 cases in that battle alone (Shepherd, 2000). As well as being treated at the front, many were shipped back to the UK. For the rank and file the army established Maghull, which drew together a specialist team of 67 medical officers to try "the psychological ideas of Dejerine, Janet and Freud" (Shepherd, 2000).

At Maghull, W. H. R. Rivers found that the patients confirmed Freud's theories that "dreams have the fulfilment of a wish as their motive" (Rivers, 1932), and then he moved on to Craiglockhart Hospital, where he treated Siegfried Sassoon and became "the most interesting of the shell-shock doctors" (Shepherd, 2000).

The experience of treating shell-shock led Rivers to recognise the value and wide application of Freud's theory of the unconscious, but to categorically disagree with the notion that all neurosis was produced by sexual factors, stating that with shell-shock it relates "directly, to the strains and shocks of warfare" (Rivers, 1917). By the end of the war, Freud too had revised his theories to encompass a model of what happens in trauma, where dreams can be seen as "helping carry out another task" which is to "master the stimulus retrospectively" (Freud, 1920).

The First World War can be regarded as a crucible for the testing of psychoanalytic theories and by the end of it, the British medical establishment begrudgingly gave some degree of credibility to psychological medicine.

Grace Pailthorpe was one of the British doctors who served during WW1.

She had begun her career in medicine at the London (Royal Free Hospital) School of Medicine for Women in 1908 (Montanaro, 2010) with the aim of becoming a surgeon. At that time, the usual routes for becoming a surgeon, such as taking the Tripos in Sciences at Cambridge and then attending medical school, simply were not available to women. In 1908, women did not have full access to higher education. Although women were allowed to study at university, they were not allowed to qualify in any degrees. For example, Oxford did not start giving degrees to women until 1920 and Cambridge did not award women degrees until 1948. Pailthorpe qualified in 1914 (Montanaro, 2010), at the outbreak of the First World War and decided to volunteer.

She went to the War Office in London and filled in her application but was rejected on grounds of her sex (Pailthorpe, 1914–19). In her journal, she wrote: "Leaving the War Office, sadly, once more with the brutal way in which one's sex was utilised by the ruling sex to domineer. I made my way to every hospital unit that I heard about asking to be allowed to 'join up'. One after the other told me either that they weren't taking women or, in the case of women's hospitals that they already had a long list and they would add my name" (Pailthorpe, 1914–19).

Where no opportunity existed, she created her own by side-stepping the British establishment and volunteering with the French Red Cross. Here, she worked at the Bromley-Martin Hospital Unit in the Haute-Marne District in France. This hospital had been set up by Madeline Bromley-Martin, a minor member of the nobility, in a chateau 60 miles behind the lines (Gladstone, 2017). The chief surgeon was Dr Graham Aspland (a gynaecologist) and the anaesthetist was Henry Tonks, the painter and Slade Art School Professor (Gladstone, 2017). It had a staff of 60 and 110 beds to serve the wounded from the French 3rd Army Corps (Gladstone, 2017).

At the Bromley-Martin she saw the brutality of war first-hand.

In her autobiographical notes she describes removing the bandages of a patient who had been labelled "scalp wound" to find that "a good size piece of his skull had been blown away and received a considerable portion of his brain tissue into my hand" (Pailthorpe, 1914–18). On another occasion they opened a man's chest and "blood shot to the ceiling" (Pailthorpe, 1914–18) from an aneurism. The surgeon froze and she had to spring past him and clamp the artery with her hand to save the man's life.

Pailthorpe showed much frustration with the British medical establishment and by the end of the war realised that she would never have the opportunity to become the surgeon that she wanted to be. However, during World War 1, she had developed an interest in psychological medicine, and in 1922 (Walsh, 1998), she began training at the London Institute of Psychoanalysis (Nölleke, 2007–2023) under Ernest Jones (Stefana & Montanaro, 2023; Walsh, 1998). The latter was a key figure in British psychoanalysis. He was a close confidante of Freud. It was also Jones who later helped Freud to escape from the Nazis to London on the eve of World War 2.

In 1923, Pailthorpe additionally started working with Maurice Hamblin Smith, who was Britain's first authorised "criminologist" (Garland, 1988; Shapira, 2013), and a lecturer on criminology at the University of Birmingham and Bethlem Royal Hospital, London. Smith (1922) believed that getting into "the mind of the offender" was essential to understanding crime and "solving the problem of delinquency." The work that Pailthorpe would do with Smith led to the birth of a psychoanalytic criminology and a paradigm shift in the way of thinking about crime and criminology.

After World War 1 a new emphasis on the clinical examination of offenders had emerged from the work of the French psychologist Alfred Binet, who in 1904 had developed a test for identifying the "feeble minded"

(Rose, 1989). Between 1908 and 1911, he revised his work transforming it from a technique for diagnosing the pathological into a scale for mapping the normal (Shapira, 2013). In Britain, this work was adapted by Cyril Burt to give rise to psychometric testing, through which the previously ungraspable domain of mental capacities was opened up into numbers, quotients, and scores that could be turned into profiles that made the individual knowable (Shapira, 2013).

This was one of the new theoretical tools that Pailthorpe was to use in 1922 for her study of women offenders (Saville, 1992; Walsh, 1998). As so often in her life, this seems to have come about because she took the initiative and, when an opportunity did not exist, created it.

At that time only a few psychoanalysts had begun to develop psycho-analytic thinking in relation to the field of criminality (Ruszczynski, 2016). Freud had written "Criminals from a sense of guilt" in 1916 and later Melanie Klein would also add to the literature on the subject by writing "Criminal tendencies in normal children" (1927) and "On criminality" (1934).

It was on the strength of this line of research that Pailthorpe established the Institute for the Scientific Treatment of Delinquency (ISTD) in 1931. The stated aim of the ISTD was to find a better way to treat criminals, based on scientific research (ISTD, 1934). Her ambition was that treatment might replace punishment. To further this aim in 1933 the ISTD established a clinical wing—the Psychopathic Clinic. The Clinic was born between the two great wars, during a particularly stormy period of history which saw the birth of Communism, the rise of National Socialism, civil unrest across Europe (including the Spanish Civil War), economic collapse, and the Great Depression.

Pailthorpe's ideas around criminology were not widely popular as they went against both right and left wing thinking of the time. The right wanted to emphasise the rule of law and punish criminals, while the left, as represented by the Fabian movement and the incipient Labour Party, wanted to locate the causes of crime in poverty and the social injustices of the economic system. A psychoanalytic approach such as Pailthorpe's, which locates the causes of crime within the individual, did not, and still does not, fit easily within the adversarial party politics of Britain.

Pailthorpe's journey to Surrealism came about like the chance meeting of a sewing machine and an umbrella on a dissecting table when, in 1935, while attending a party given by the minor poet and literary critic Victor Neuberg (who had also acted as secretary in the setting up of the ISTD), she met the artist Reuben Mednikoff. They locked eyes, discussed the subconscious and how art could be used as a means of curing mental problems, oblivious of the party going on around them as it degenerated into fin de siècle debauchery. It was not so much love at first sight as a recognition that together they could pursue the scientific experiments they were interested in carrying out.

Pailthorpe's background and her approach to Surrealism marked her as different from the other artists, but she got on well with Andre Breton, who acknowledged her and Reuben Mednikoff, as "the best and most truly surrealist" of the British artists. It might be their similar history and clinical experience in World War 1 that helped them connect. Andre Breton had been in the French Medical Corps and had worked at a number of hospitals, caring for shell shock patients. Although he never qualified, he trained in psychiatry, neurology and even spent a while working under Babinski at *La Pitié* in Paris (Polizzotti, 1955).

It has been said that there are two Surrealisms. The first is the one that pushes art beyond the realism of the nineteenth century so that it manifests a strange reality imbued with the psychological projections of the unconscious mind. This is the Surrealism that is best known from the paintings of Salvador Dali and Rene Magritte. The second is the Surrealism that finds surreal elements through an intensely close examination of reality. This is the Surrealism of Georges Franju's film "La Sange des Betes" or the extra-ordinary anthropological and sociological work of Georges Bataille and his Acéphale group, which explored subjects such as scatology, death and the erotic, base materialism, and the aesthetics of the formless.

Pailthorpe managed to straddle both kinds of Surrealism—the first in the dream-obsessed, sexual, scatological, and "Freudian"[3] images of her paintings and the second in her meticulous and detailed analysis of both her and Reuben Mednikoff's work.

Surrealism has remained very much a European movement and only a minor part of the British artistic tradition. Britain acknowledged surrealist painting, but never really engaged with the wider intellectual and literary traditions of Surrealism. Important surrealist thinkers and writers of the "anti-tradition" such as Alfred Jarry, Louis Aragon, Robert Desnos, Walter Serner, and George Bataille remain relatively unknown here. Similarly, from a European perspective, the British contribution to Surrealism scarcely rises to the level of a footnote.

Within the art world, Pailthorpe's work has been very much on the margins. The same is true of psychoanalysis (Stefana & Montanaro, 2023).

Psychoanalysis, in many ways, was quite a conservative discipline and so, despite the surrealist interest in the unconscious, psychoanalysis as a discipline did not really engage with Surrealism. Surrealism courted scandal and publicity at a time when psychoanalysis was attempting to put itself on a scientific footing and trying to project a professional image. Pailthorpe's involvement with Surrealism would almost certainly have marginalised her within the psychoanalytic community.

Pailthorpe's life took place at many contested intersections: she was the only daughter in a family of boys, a woman trying to become a surgeon, a scientist exploring art, and positioned herself on behalf of the criminal. She was often categorised as awkward and difficult to get along with, but in fact she simply did not fit into the categories that she was offered and was unwilling to quietly accept how things were. Where she did not find opportunities available, she made her own and kicked against the unjust application of power. This is something that seems to have run through her entire life.

Her work, and that of the Portman Clinic, with criminals also occurs at a highly contested intersection of discourses. Criminals are a highly minoritised[4] group that society prefers to lock away and forget about. Criminals are Othered as a group that conducts acts, behaviours, and thoughts that society cannot acknowledge in itself, so criminals are frequently positioned as needing to be punished and be rid of. Alternative discourses about how to treat prisoners are also often regarded with suspicion and called "soft," while society rarely reflects on the sadistic element of its desire to punish.

This desire to punish without understanding re-enacts the "event" of the criminal act itself. It forecloses the possibility of the painstaking work of understanding through, often evacuative and sometimes impulsive, action.

Although her paintings and writings form one part of Pailthorpe's legacy, she also created a living legacy in the Portman Clinic through the work of the many clinicians who have followed in her footsteps and the patients who have benefitted. The Portman Clinic saw its first patient in 1933 and since then has seen over 20,000 individuals for assessment or treatment.

There is a strange attraction between the liberatory politics of Surrealism that Pailthorpe engaged with in her surrealist painting and writing, and the somewhat more pragmatic and practical approach of the Portman in helping the least free in society, attempting to liberate its patients from a past that often drives them into the physically containing (and psychically uncharted) environment of prison.

In many ways, there must be something pragmatic and practical about a setting such as the Portman Clinic, which deals with unsettling and disturbing and disturbed states of mind. Prison is the ultimate—concrete—setting to manage such patients, but many could (and many of those who have the opportunity to come to the Portman, do) benefit from having the curious mind of the clinician within a secure physical setting. For the Portman's patients, a curious (parental) mind was often not available in their neglected, violent, and disturbed upbringings. And in this sense, the "Portman building" itself can be understood as being a fundamental part of the therapeutic provision.

The Portman Clinic was created to examine the fringes of society. Founded during the political and social upheaval of the interwar years, it dealt with those thrown up and then tossed aside by a turbulent world. From its inception, the Portman Clinic has had as its purpose: assessment, treatment, and research (ISTD, 1934). It seeks to understand the unconscious motivations that drive certain offending behaviours. It places each crime not only in the context of its details, but also looks at the whole person within an environment.

Just as the criminal act can place the offender outside society, so can the artistic techniques of the surrealists place their images outside reality. As a group the surrealists also positioned themselves beyond society, attacking bourgeoise mentality and hypocritical morality. Society does the reverse with criminals.

The criminal act is understandable in one sense as an action against society, but it is also unconsciously a self-destructive act, which harms the offender (not only literally, but also the offender's internal objects— important and dependable figures in the offender's own unconscious mind). Criminal behaviour can be explosive, violent, or uncontrollable. It can be the equivalent of a neurotic symptom, a sign of personality disorder, or just plain criminality.

The experience of working with forensic cases, over almost 90 years, shows that punishing criminals neither helps the criminal nor protects society. As Stanley Ruszczynski, a former Director of the Portman Clinic, said, "Our patients grow up in hell, and then they carry out hellish acts, and we respond as a society by putting them into hell, with the expectation that they'll come out and become un-hellish" (Sarner, 2022).

Prisons are expensive and ineffective as tools for the prevention of crime or reforming prisoners. The fact that they still exist suggests that the function that prisons actually perform is located elsewhere. The futility and expense of punishing criminals serve the purpose of gratifying and comforting the wider public, allowing society to exercise its sadistic drives while at the same time, through the process of projective identification, locating aggressive impulses in the criminal "other."

Forensic psychotherapy has found that society is also to a degree complicit in the psychodrama of criminal behaviour. As well as vicariously enjoying the enactment of its own unconscious forbidden desires, society provides an audience that takes pleasure in indulging its own anger and outrage. The culture of blame can be likened to the primitive defence mechanisms of splitting and projective identification that see people in the black and white terms of good and evil. Society protects the self-image of its own goodness by projecting badness into others and such group dynamics and social fantasies can be incredibly powerful.

The psychoanalytic orientation of the Portman Clinic goes back to its origins and over the years has evolved to include not only the original Freudian orientation but also theory and practice stemming from Klein (and her followers), and from the Independent school.

The disturbed and disturbing behaviour of criminals (and other patients) is understood as a way of communicating or dealing with unprocessed internal states. A key insight of the Portman Clinic's approach is to bear in mind that the patient is both victim and perpetrator—but to neither collude with the first nor to demonise and condemn the latter.

The approach is not to condone the crime or excuse the criminal. Instead, the aim is to help the offender acknowledge responsibility for their acts.

Violence and other disordered acts can often be traced back to similar events that occurred in childhood. Every perpetrator has also already been a victim. It is a tenet of the Portman Clinic that such acts are potentially preventable and the emotional states that cause them are treatable, liberating the patient from the prison of their past.

Nowadays, the Portman Clinic practises what it calls "forensic psychotherapy," a detailed, long-term treatment designed to help those who have nowhere else to go but back to jail. It is a relatively recently created discipline that applies psychoanalytic knowledge to the assessment, management, and treatment of mentally disordered offenders, forming a bridge between traditional forensic psychiatry—with its focus on diagnosis and risk—and traditional psychotherapy—with its focus on understanding why things happen, why things have happened, and why they will happen again in the future.

Although forensic psychotherapy may seem like a narrow field, as with other areas of medicine an understanding of illness also contributes more widely to an understanding of health. By looking at the outliers of society the Portman Clinic has deepened the understanding of the totality of human behaviour. With the accumulation of substantial clinical experience, the initial idealism of Pailthorpe has been modified and has evolved into something more realistic and perhaps more hopeful.

Portman clinicians treat individuals with complicated and severe psychopathologies, believing that, as long as unconscious motives are disregarded, it is impossible to learn more about crime than common sense tells us. As with Jarry's pataphysics, you cannot understand the exception to the rule by looking at the rule. Common sense is not enough to understand the fundamental flight from reality that leads to pathological behaviour. This understanding of the disavowal of reality at the heart of much perverse, violent, and delinquent behaviour places what is, in many ways, a surreal concept at the core of contemporary clinical practice in the Portman Clinic today.

Grace Pailthope's interest in surreal art is mirrored, like the double image of a Salvador Dali painting, by the Portman Clinic's "psychoanalytic interest" in the sporadically irrational, bizarre, unconventional nature and behaviour of its patients: the violence, perversity, delinquency … and also behaviour which is sometimes difficult and disturbing to hear about. There is often something disconcerting about the forensic Portman patient, just as there is about much surreal art. The meanings are complex, multi-layered, deliberately ambiguous, and often subversively provocative. There is frequently an element of shock. You can see "the reality," but there is always more to it.

Glenn Gossling
February 2023

Notes

1 The Portman Clinic, part of the Tavistock and Portman NHS Foundation Trust, is a National Health Service (NHS) specialist forensic psychotherapy out-patient clinic offering assessment, treatment, and consultation services for adults, children, and adolescents troubled by problems of criminality, violence, sexual difficulties, or antisocial personality disorder.

2 The first abridged translation of Freud's *The Interpretation of Dreams* was *On Dreams* by James Stratchey and had been published in 1901 by the Hogarth Press.
3 At that time Psychoanalysis was quite strictly Freudian. Anyone who diverged too far from Freudian orthodoxy was expelled, as happened with Alfred Adler in 1911, Carl Jung in 1913 and Wilhelm Reich in 1934. Grace Pailthorpe trained under Ernest Jones during the 1920s. Jones was close to Freud, but was also influenced by Melanie Klein as were many British analysts of the time. The schism between Kleinian and Freudian thinking had not yet emerged and both Jones and Klein viewed Klein's ideas as part of Freudian analysis. Grace Pailthorpe viewed herself as Freudian, but also acknowledged Klein as an influence. However, as Alberto Stefana (2018, 2019) asserts, looking back retrospectively Pailthorpe more properly stands in a line of European thought that starts with *The Interpretation of Dreams* and passes through Surrealism.
4 "Minorité" is a philosophical concept developed by Gilles Deleuze and Félix Guattari in their books Kafka: *Towards a Minor Literature* (1975) and *A Thousand Plateaus* (1980), and as a concept is in opposition to the majoritarian "state machine."

References

Crichton-Miller, H. (1933). *Psycho-analysis and its derivatives*. Home University Library.
Crichton-Miller, H. (1961). *Hugh Crichton-Miller 1877–1959, A personal memoir*. Friary Press.
Freud, S. (1920). Beyond the pleasure principle. *Standard Edition, 18*, 7–64.
Garland, D. (1988). British criminology before 1935. *British Journal of Criminology, 28*(2), 1–17.
Gladstone, M. (2017). Converting a royal residence into a functional hospital presented a challenge. *The Courier and Advertiser (Perth and Perthshire Edition)*, 6 June.
Hamblin Smith, M. (1922). *The psychology of the criminal*. Methuen.
ISTD (1934). *Institute for the Scientific Treatment of Delinquency Report for the year ended December 31st, 1933*. ISTD.
Jenkins, W. J. (2017). *An analysis of Sigmund Freud's The Interpretation of Dreams*. Macat Library.
Jones, E. (1910). Freud's theory of dreams. *The American Journal of Psychology, 21*(2), 283–308.
Kahr, B. (2018). *New horizons in forensic psychotherapy: Exploring the work of Estela V. Welldon*. Routledge
Montanaro, L. A. (2010). *Surrealism and psychoanalysis in the work of Grace Pailthorpe and Reuben Mednikoff: 1935–1940*. University of Edinburgh.
Myers, C. S. (1915). A contribution to the study of shell shock. *Lancet, 185*(4772), 316–320.
Nölleke, B. (2007–2023). Grace W. Pailthorpe (1883–1971). Psychoanalytikerinnen, Biografisches Lexikon. https://www.psychoanalytikerinnen.de/greatbritain_biographies.html#Pailthorpe
Pailthorpe, G. (1914–18). Diary notes by Pailthorpe on 'the war period', dated 04.08.14. Scottish National Gallery of Modern Art Archive (File 25 'Wartime file titled: 'Doc in First World War 1914–1918''), 1.
Pailthorpe, G. (1914–18). 1914–1918 wartime file titled: 'Doc in First World War 1914–1918', Scottish National Gallery of Modern Art Archive, GMA A62.
Pailthorpe, G. (1938–39). The scientific aspect of Surrealism. In A. Stefana & L. A. Montanaro (Eds.), *Grace Pailthorpe's writings on psychoanalysis and Surrealism* (pp. 53–61). Routledge, 2023.

Polizzotti, M. (1955). *Revolution of the mind. The life of Andre Breton*. Bloomsbury.

Rivers, W. H. R. (1917). Freud's psychology of the unconscious. *Lancet*, *189*(4894), 912–914.

Rivers, W. H. R. (1932). *Conflict and dream*. Routledge, 2001.

Rose, N. (1989). *Governing the soul*. Routledge.

Ruszczynski, S. (2016). A brief introduction to the history of the Portman Clinic. *Journal of Child Psychotherapy*, *42*(3), 262–265.

Sarner, M. (2022). A ninety-year history of the Portman Clinic. *International Journal of Forensic Psychotherapy*, *4*(1), 12–20.

Saville, E. (1992). *Let justice be done*. ISTD.

Shapira, M. (2013). *The war inside*. Cambridge University Press.

Shepherd, B. (2000). *War of nerves*. Jonathan Cape.

Stefana, A. (2018). From *Die Traumdeutung* to *The Squiggle Game*: A brief history of an evolution. *American Journal of Psychoanalysis*, *78*(2), 182–194.

Stefana, A. (2019). Revisiting Marion Milner's work on creativity and art. *International Journal of Psychoanalysis*, *100*(1), 128–147.

Stefana, A., & Montanaro, L. A. (2023). Introduction. In *Grace Pailthorpe's writings on psychoanalysis and Surrealism*. Routledge.

Stratchey, J. (1901). *On dreams*. Hogarth Press

Walsh, N., & Wilson, A. (1998). *Sluice Gates of the mind*. Leeds Museums and Galleries.

Woolf, V. (1924). *Mr. Bennett and Mrs. Brown*. Hogarth Press.

References

Anzieu, D. (1975). *Freud's self-analysis*. Hogarth Press.

Aronson, M. (1980). Geographical and socioeconomic factors in the 1881 anti-Jewish pogroms in Russia. *Russian Review*, *39*(1), 18–31.

Author Unknown. (1933). Today's art: Fashion in painting. *Sunday Referee*, May 21.

Author Unknown. (1934). Criminal and social problems in Kenya. In an unnamed newspaper, March 27. Edinburgh: Dean Gallery Archive, File 29.

Author Unknown. (1969). Exhibition of recent paintings by Dr. Grace W. Pailthorpe. *The President's New Bulletin*, *15*(2).

Bacciagaluppi, M. (2017). Pierre Janet and Auguste Forel: Two historical contributions. *American Journal of Psychoanalysis*, *77*, 417–439.

Bacopoulos-Viau, A. (2012). Automatism, Surrealism and the making of French psychopathology: The case of Pierre Janet. *History of Psychiatry*, *23*(3), 259–276.

Becker, A. (2000). The avant-garde, madness and the great war. *Journal of Contemporary History*, *35*(1), 71–84.

Blum, H. P. (2017). Tribute to Graziella Magherini. Freud's travels and the Stendhal Syndrome. *PsicoArt*, 7.

Bogue, A. (1940). *Correspondence with Pailthorpe concerning the USA*. Unpublished manuscript. Scottish National Gallery of Modern Art, A62/1/006.

Breton, A. (1924). *Manifestes Du Surréalisme*. University of Michigan Press.

Breton, A. (1937–40). *Correspondences on Surrealism in Britain*. Unpublished manuscript. Scottish National Gallery of Modern Art, A62/1/102.

Breton, A. (1941). Artistic genesis and perspective of Surrealism. In *Surrealism and painting* (pp. 49–82). MacDonald, 1972.

Breton, A. (1967). Visite à Leon Trotsky. In *La Clé des champs* (p. 55). Jean-Jacques Pauvert.

Breton, A., & Rivera, D. (1938–39). Towards an independent revolutionary art. *London Bulletin*, 7 (pp.29–32).

Breton, A., & Soupault, P. (1920). *Les Champs magnétiques. Suivi de S'Il vous plaît et de Vous m'oublierez*. Gallimard.

Breton, A., & Trotsky, L. (1938). *Pour un art révolutionnaire indépendant* (I. Henderson, Trans.). Scottish National Gallery of Modern Art.

Breuer, J., & Freud, S. (1892–95). *Studies on hysteria*, vol. 2. Hogarth.

Brierley, M. (1933). General: Anon. 'Psychology of delinquency.' British Medical Journal, October 29th, 1932, p. 801. *International Journal of Psycho-Analysis*, *14*, 109.

Buck, L. (1988). *The surrealist spirit in Britain*. Whitford & Hughes.

Cassullo, G. (2019). Freud meets Janet: Notes towards a psychology of the Plural-Ego. *Italian Psychoanalytic Annual*, *13*, 99–116.

Chevrier A. (2001). André Breton et la psychopathologie de son temps: deux exemples [André Breton and the psychopathology of his time: Two examples]. In *Mélusine, Cahiers du Centre de recherche sur le surré alisme, XXI. Réalisme-surré alisme* (pp. 213–226). Éditions l'À ge d'Homme.

Chilvers, I., & Glaves-Smith, J. (2009). *A dictionary of modern and contemporary art.* Second edition. Oxford University Press.

Collins, C. (1940). *Letter to Mednikoff on the Barcelona meeting.* Unpublished manuscript. Scottish National Gallery of Modern Art, A62/1/108.

Colquhoun, I. (1940). *Correspondences on the Stafford Gallery exhibition.* Unpublished manuscript. Scottish National Gallery of Modern Art, A62/1/112.

Colquhoun, I. (1940). *Letters to Mednikoff on the Barcelona meeting.* Unpublished manuscript. Scottish National Gallery of Modern Art, A62/1/108.

Cordess, C. (1992). Pioneers in forensic psychiatry. Edward Glover (1888–1972): Psychoanalysis and crime – A fragile legacy. *Journal of Forensic Psychiatry & Psychology, 3*, 509–530.

Crabtree, A. (2003). 'Automatism' and the emergence of dynamic psychiatry. *Journal of the History of the Behavioral Sciences, 39*(1), 51–70.

Dearborn, M. (2006). *Peggy Guggenheim: Mistress of modernism.* Virago Press.

Dimsdale, C. (n.d.). *Correspondences.* Unpublished manuscript. Scottish National Gallery of Modern Art, A62/1/183.

Ellenberger, H. F. (1970). *The discovery of the unconscious.* New Basic Books.

Esman, A. H. (2011). Psychoanalysis and Surrealism: André Breton and Sigmund Freud. *Journal of the American Psychoanalytic Association, 59*, 173–181. 10.1177/0003065111403146.

Fenichel, O. (1939). Pailthorpe, Grace W.: The analysis of a poem. *International Journal of Psycho-Analysis, 19*(2), 352.

Ferenczi, S. (1932). *The clinical diary of Sándor Ferenczi.* Harvard University Press, 1988.

Fischer Fine Art Limited. (1976). *Conroy Maddox, Gouaches of the 1940's.* Fischer Fine Art Ltd.

Flugel, J., & West, D. (1933). *A hundred years of Psychology 1833–1933.* Gerald Duckworth & Co. Ltd.

Fordham, M. (1978). *Jungian psychotherapy. A study in analytical psychology.* John Wiley & Sons.

Freud, S. (1896a). *Heredity and the aetiology of the neuroses*, vol. 3. Hogarth.

Freud, S. (1896b). *Further remarks on the neuropsychoses of defence*, vol. 3. Hogarth.

Freud, S. (1896c). *The aetiology of hysteria*, vol 3. Hogarth.

Freud, S. (1899). *The interpretation of dreams*, vols. 4 and 5. Hogarth.

Freud, S. (1906). Delusions and dreams in Jensen's Gradiva. *SE, 9*, 3–95.

Freud, S. (1910). Leonardo da Vinci and a memory of his childhood. *SE, 11*, 59–137.

Freud, S. (1912). Recommendations to physicians practising psycho-analysis. *SE, 12.*

Freud, S. (1913). On beginning the treatment (Further recommendations on the technique of psychoanalysis I). *SE, 12*, 121–144.

Freud, S. (1919). Lines of advance in psycho-analytic therapy. *SE, 17*, 159–168.

Freud, S. (1929). Civilization and its discontents. *SE, 21*, 57–146.

Gamba, A., & Stefana, A. (2016). "Sono innamor(a)to della terra." Note su gioco, disegno, sogno e terapie diversionali nella cura di bambini con gravi patologie fisiche. *Psicoterapia e Scienze Umane, 50*(2), 207–228.

Gamba, A., & Stefana, A. (2023). Making the best in a bad job: A psychoanalytic perspective on communication with children and adolescents with severe physical conditions. *Psychoanalytic Quarterly, 92*(3), 463–497.

Garland, D. (2002). Of crimes and criminals: The development of criminology in Britain. In M. Maguire, R. Morgan, & R. Reiner (Eds.), *The Oxford handbook of criminology* (3rd ed.). Oxford University Press.

Gascoyne, D. (1936). *Correspondence with Reuben Mednikoff.* Unpublished manuscript. Scottish National Gallery of Modern Art.

Glover, E. (1933). What we put in prison: By G. W. Pailthorpe, M.D. (Williams & Norgate, London, 1932. Pp. 159. Price 5s. net.). *International Journal of Psycho-Analysis, 14*, 278–279.

Glover, N. (2009). *Psychoanalytic aesthetics: An introduction to the British School.* Karnac.

Gordon, R. G. (1928). *Autolycus or the future for miscreant youth.* K. Paul, Trench, Trubner & Company.

Haan, J., Koehler, P. J., & Bogousslavsky, J. (2012). Neurology and Surrealism: André Breton and Joseph Babinski. *Brain, 135*(12), 3830–3838.

Halliday Faux, N. (2003). *More than a bookshop: Zwemmer's and art in the 20th century.* Philip Wilson Publishers.

Hamblin Smith, M. (1922). *The psychology of the criminal.* Methuen.

Hamblin Smith, M., & Pailthorpe, G. W. (1923). Mental tests for delinquents, and mental conflict as a cause of delinquency. *Lancet, 2*, 112–114.

Hampstead Artists' Council. (1975). *Hampstead in the thirties: A committed decade [Exhibition catalog].* Arkwright Arts Trust.

Harrison, C. (1981). *English art and modernism 1900–1939.* Yale University Press.

Isaacs, S. (1952). The nature and function of phantasy. In M.Klein *Developments in psychoanalysis* (Eds.), (pp. 67–121). London: Hogarth Press.

Janet, P. (1889). *L'automatisme psychologique: Essai de psychologie expérimentale sur les formes inférieures de l'activité humaine.* Félix Alcan.

Janet, P. (1890). *L'automatisme psychologique.* Felix Alcan.

Jensen, E. T. (1940). *Letter to an unknown organisation on Pailthorpe's move to the USA.* Unpublished manuscript. Scottish National Gallery of Modern Art, A62/1/003.

Jones, D. W. (2016). *Disordered personalities and crime.* Routledge.

Jones, E. (1914–15). Professor Janet on psychoanalysis: A rejoinder. *Journal of Abnormal Psychology, 9*, 400–410.

Jung, C. G. (1906). *Diagnostische Assoziationsstudien: Beiträge zur experimentellen Psychopathologie [Diagnosticassociation studies: contributions to experimental psychopathology]*, vol. 1. Verlag von Johann Ambrosius.

Jung, C. G. (1913–1930). In S. Shamdasani (Ed.), *The red book: Liber novus.* W. W. Norton & Company, 2009.

Jung, C. G. (1921). Psychological types. *Collected works of C.G. Jung, Vol. 6: Psychological types.* Pantheon Books, 1971.

Jung, C. G. (1929). The aims of psychotherapy. *Collected works of C.G. Jung, Vol. 16: Practice of psychotherapy.* Pantheon Books, 1977.

Jung, C. G. (1934). The meaning of psychology for modern man. *Collected works of C.G. Jung, Vol. 10: Civilization in transition.* Princeton University Press, 1970.

Jung, C. G. (1936). Psychological factors determining human behavior. *Collected works of C.G. Jung, Vol. 8: The structure and dynamics of the psyche.* Princeton University Press, 1978.

Jung, C. G. (1961). *Memories, dreams, reflections.* Collins and Routledge.

Kahr, B. (2018). *New horizons in forensic psychotherapy: Exploring the work of Estela V. Welldon.* Routledge.

Kaplan, D. M. (1989). Surrealism and psychoanalysis: Notes on a cultural affair. *American Imago, 6*, 319–327.

Klein, M. (1923). The development of a child. *International Journal of Psycho-Analysis, 4*, 419–474.

Klein, M. (1926). Infant analysis. *International Journal of Psycho-Analysis, 7*, 31–63.

Klein, M. (1926). The psychological principles of infant analysis. *International Journal of Psychoanalysis, 8*, 25–37.

Klein, M. (1927). Symposium on child-analysis. *International Journal of Psycho-Analysis, 8*, 339–370.

Klein, M. (1929). Personification in the play of children. *International Journal of Psycho-Analysis, 10*, 193–204.

Klein, M. (1932). *The psycho-analysis of children.* Hogarth Press.

Klein, M. (1935). A contribution to the psychogenesis of manic-depressive states. *International Journal of Psychoanalysis, 16*, 145–174.

Klein, M. (1948). A contribution to the theory of anxiety and guilt. *International Journal of Psychoanalysis, 29*, 114–123.

Klein, M. (1957). Envy and gratitude. In M. Klein (Eds.), *Envy and gratitude and other works 1946–1963. The writings of Melanie Klein (vol. III).* The Hogarth Press and the Institute of Psycho-Analysis.

Klein, M. (1959). Our adult world and its roots in infancy. In *Our adult world and other essays.* Heinemann Medical Books, 1963.

Langdon-Brown, W. (1940). *Letter to an unknown organisation on Pailthorpe's move to the USA.* Unpublished manuscript. Scottish National Gallery of Modern Art, A62/1/003.

Larocque, Y. M. (2007). Grace Pailthorpe et Reuben Mednikoff à Vancouver. La transmission du Surréalisme au Canada anglais, 1942–1946. *RACAR: revue d'art canadienne / Canadian Art Review, 32*, 35–44.

Levy, S. (2003). *The scandalous eye: The Surrealism of Conroy Maddox.* Liverpool University Press.

Lewis, H. (1988). *The politics of Surrealism.* Paragon House Publishers.

Macdonald, J. W. G. (1954). Lettre de Jock Macdonald à Margaret McLaughlin, 5 novembre 1954; Archives de la galerie McLaughlin, Oshawa, fonds J. W. G. Macdonald.

Maclagan, D. (1992). Between psychoanalysis and Surrealism: The collaboration between Grace Pailthorpe and Reuben Mednikoff. *Free Associations, 1*, 33–50.

Maclagan, D. (1998). Making for mother. In N. Walsh & A. Wilson (Eds.), *See sluice gates of the mind: The collaborative work of Pailthorpe and Mednikoff.* City Art Gallery.

Maddox, C. (n.d.). *Correspondences.* Unpublished manuscript. Scottish National Gallery of Modern Art, RPA/286.

Maddox, C., Melville, J., & Melville, R. (1940). *Letter to Mednikoff.* Unpublished manuscript. Scottish National Gallery of Modern Art, A62/1/108.

Magritte, R. (1938). In A. Blavier (Ed.), *Écrits complets.* Flammarion, 2009.

Makari, G. J. (1997). Dora's hysteria and the maturation of Sigmund Freud's transference theory: A new historical interpretation. *Journal of the American Psychoanalytic Association, 45*(4), 1061–1096.

Martel, G. (Ed.). (1999). *The origins of the Second World War reconsidered.* Routledge.

McWilliam, F. (1940). *Letter to Mednikoff on the Barcelona meeting.* Unpublished manuscript. Scottish National Gallery of Modern Art, A62/1/108.

Mednikoff, R. (1930–70). *Personal file.* Unpublished manuscript. Scottish National Gallery of Modern Art, A62/1/062.

Mednikoff, R. (1935). *Extracts from diary.* Unpublished manuscript. Scottish National Gallery of Modern Art, A62/1/019.

Mednikoff, R. (1935a). *Diary extracts.* Unpublished manuscript. Tate Britain Gallery Archives.

Mednikoff, R. (1935b). *Correspondence with David Gascoyne.* Unpublished manuscript. Scottish National Gallery of Modern Art.

Mednikoff, R. (1940). *Letters to the Surrealist group.* Unpublished manuscript. Scottish National Gallery of Modern Art, A62/1/108.

Mertens, W. (1999).*Traum und Traumdeutung [Dream and interpretation of dreams]*. Beck.

Mertens, W. (2000). L'interpretazione dei sogni cento anni dopo [The interpretation of dreams, one hundred years later]. *Psicoterapia e Scienze Uman, XXXIV*, 5–30.

Mesens, E. L. T. (n.d.). *Correspondences*. Unpublished manuscript. Scottish National Gallery of Modern Art, RPA/708.

Mesens, E. L. T. (1934). L'Action Immédiate. *Documents, 34*, 8.

Mesens, E. L. T. (1940). *Declaration to Surrealist group*. Unpublished manuscript. Scottish National Gallery of Modern Art, RPA/722.

Milner, M. (1950). *On not being able to paint*. Routledge, 2010.

Montanaro, L. A. (2010). *Surrealism and psychoanalysis in the work of Grace Pailthorpe and Reuben Mednikoff: 1935–1940* (Doctoral dissertation, The University of Edinburgh). Available online at: http://www.artcornwall.org/features/Pailthorpe_Mednikoff.pdf

Nadeau, M. (1968). *The history of Surrealism*. Cape.

Neuberg, V. E. (1983). *Vickybird: A memoir of Victor B. Neuberg*. London Polytechnic.

Overy, R. (1994). *Inter-war crisis 1919–1939*. Longman

Pailthorpe, G. W. (1914–18). *'Document in First World War'*. Unpublished manuscript. Scottish National Gallery of Modern Art, A62/1/025.

Pailthorpe, G. W. (1914–22). *Autobiographical notes (re 'Kid')*. Unpublished manuscript. Scottish National Gallery of Modern Art, A62/1/081.

Pailthorpe, G. W. (1920–22). *Travel autobiography 'Truants'*. Unpublished manuscript. Scottish National Gallery of Modern Art, A62/1/046.

Pailthorpe, G. W. (1920–29). *Autobiographical notes (re Bob); Text on legality of punishment and legal processes*. Unpublished manuscript. Scottish National Gallery of Modern Art, A62/1/078.

Pailthorpe, G. W. (1921). *Diary of South Sea Island Trip*. Unpublished manuscript. Scottish National Gallery of Modern Art, A62/1/028.

Pailthorpe, G. W. (1923). *Pailthorpe's scheme for prison research*. Unpublished manuscript. Scottish National Gallery of Modern Art, A62/1/060.

Pailthorpe, G. W. (1925). *Beginning of autobiography*. Unpublished manuscript. Scottish National Gallery of Modern Art, A62/1/152.

Pailthorpe, G. W. (1926–27). *Typescript 'Report on a psychological investigation of the inmates of preventive & rescue homes in London 1926–27' and accompanying correspondence*. Unpublished manuscript. Scottish National Gallery of Modern Art, A62/1/007.

Pailthorpe, G. W. (1928–34). *Document: 'Institute for the Scientific Treatment of Delinquency'*. Unpublished manuscript. Scottish National Gallery of Modern Art, A62/1/169.

Pailthorpe, G. W. (1930). *Press cuttings ('What we put in prison') of South Africa*. Unpublished manuscript. Scottish National Gallery of Modern Art, A62/1/029.

Pailthorpe, G. W. (1932a). *Studies in the psychology of delinquency*. Medical Research Council.

Pailthorpe, G. W. (1932b). *What we put in prison and in preventative and rescue homes*. Williams and Norgate.

Pailthorpe, G. W. (1932c). *Ernest Jones correspondence*. Unpublished manuscript. Scottish National Gallery of Modern Art, A62/1/001.

Pailthorpe, G. W. (1932d). *News cuttings Book 1*. Unpublished manuscript. Scottish National Gallery of Modern Art, A62/1/075.

Pailthorpe, G. W. (1932–42). *News cuttings, receipts, miscellaneous documents*. Unpublished manuscript. Scottish National Gallery of Modern Art, A62/1/165.

Pailthorpe, G. W. (1933). *Report: 'What we put in prison'.* Unpublished manuscript. Scottish National Gallery of Modern Art, A62/1/072.

Pailthorpe, G. W. (1935a). *Notes on colour symbolism.* Unpublished manuscript. Scottish National Gallery of Modern Art, A62/1/036.

Pailthorpe, G. W. (1935b). *Poems, diary and correspondence with Pailthorpe 1935–1937 (Typescript of memoir).* Tate Britain Archive (TAM 75).

Pailthorpe, G. W. (1935c). *Analytic procedure.* Unpublished manuscript. Scottish National Gallery of Modern Art, A62/1/022.

Pailthorpe, G. W. (1935–37). *Essay/texts: 'Sociological'.* Unpublished manuscript. Scottish National Gallery of Modern Art, A62/1/038.

Pailthorpe, G. W. (1935–38b).*Chronological digest of notes and drawings on Reuben Mednikoff.* Unpublished manuscript. Scottish National Gallery of Modern Art, A62/1/035.

Pailthorpe, G. W. (1935–38a). *Technique.* Unpublished manuscript. Scottish National Gallery of Modern Art, A62/1/065.

Pailthorpe, G. W. (1935–39). *Analytical observations and interpretations.* Unpublished manuscript. Scottish National Gallery of Modern Art, A62/1/138.

Pailthorpe, G. W. (1936). *Analytical notes for 'Diary' January-June.* Unpublished manuscript. Scottish National Gallery of Modern Art, A62/1/083.

Pailthorpe, G. W. (1937a). *Technique.* Unpublished manuscript. Scottish National Gallery of Modern Art, A62/1/023.

Pailthorpe, G. W. (1937b). *Analytical notes and poems.* Unpublished manuscript. Scottish National Gallery of Modern Art, A62/1/120.

Pailthorpe, G. W. (1937c). *Interpretation of paintings and drawings for public lectures, illustrated with lantern slides.* Unpublished manuscript. Scottish National Gallery of Modern Art, A62/1/014.

Pailthorpe, G. W. (1938a). The analysis of a poem. *International Journal of Psycho-Analysis, 19,* 221–225.

Pailthorpe, G. W. (1938b). *Lecture on Drawings. Being an extract from research that is now in its final stages.* Unpublished manuscript. Scottish National Gallery of Modern Art, A62/1/069.

Pailthorpe, G. W. (1938c). *'Toe dance series'.* Unpublished manuscript. Scottish National Gallery of Modern Art, A62/1/166.

Pailthorpe, G. W. (1938–39). The scientific aspect of Surrealism. *London Bulletin, 7,* 10–16. Reprinted in A. Stefana & L. A. Montanaro (Eds.), *Grace Pailthorpe's writings on psychoanalysis and Surrealism* (pp. 53–61). Routledge, 2023.

Pailthorpe, G. W. (1938–69). *Miscellaneous papers.* Unpublished manuscript. Scottish National Gallery of Modern Art, A62/1/055.

Pailthorpe, G. W. (1939). Foreword. In *Catalogue of the exhibition G. W. Pailthorpe and R. Mednikoff.* Guggenheim Jeune Gallery.

Pailthorpe, G. W. (1940). *Birth Trauma (Reuben Mednikoff).* Unpublished manuscript. Scottish National Gallery of Modern Art, A62/1/016.

Pailthorpe, G. W. (1941a). Primary processes of the infantile mind demonstrated through the analysis of a prose-poem. *International Journal of Psycho-Analysis, 22,* 44–59. Reprinted in A. Stefana & L. A. Montanaro (Eds.), *Grace Pailthorpe's writings on psychoanalysis and Surrealism* (pp. 62–64). Routledge, 2023.

Pailthorpe, G. W. (1941b). Deflection of energy, as a result of birth trauma, and its bearing upon character formation. *Psychoanalytic Review, 28,* 305–326. Reprinted in A. Stefana & L. A. Montanaro (Eds.), *Grace Pailthorpe's writings on psychoanalysis and Surrealism* (pp. 65-83). Routledge, 2023.

Pailthorpe, G. W. (1942–43). *Correspondence (various).* Unpublished manuscript. Scottish National Gallery of Modern Art, A62/1/013.

Pailthorpe, G. W. (1942–44). *Art in Canada*. Unpublished manuscript. Scottish National Gallery of Modern Art, A62/1/079.

Pailthorpe, G. W. (1944). Lecture on Surrealism. In A. Stefana & L. A. Montanaro (Eds.), *Grace Pailthorpe's writings on psychoanalysis and Surrealism* (pp. 84–90). Routledge, 2023.

Pailthorpe G. W. (1944a). Lecture on Surrealism. In A. Stefana & L. A. Montanaro (Eds.), Grace Pailthorpe's writings on psychoanalysis and Surrealism (pp. 84–90). Routledge, 2023.

Pailthorpe G. W. (1944a). Surrealism and psychology. In A. Stefana & L. A. Montanaro (Eds.), Grace Pailthorpe's writings on psychoanalysis and Surrealism (pp. 91–95). Routledge, 2023.

Pailthorpe, G. W., & Mednikoff, R. (n.d). *Draft Summary of 'Psychorealism: The Sluicegates of the emotions'*. Unpublished manuscript. Scottish National Gallery of Modern Art, A62/1/009.

Payne, S. (1944). Discussion in "Ninth Discussion of Scientific Differences". In P. King & R. Steiner (Eds.), The Freud-Klein Controversies 1941–45 (pp. 600–617). Routledge, 1991.

Payne, S. M. (1940). *Letter to an unknown organisation on Pailthorpe's move to the USA*. Unpublished manuscript. Scottish National Gallery of Modern Art, A62/1/003.

Penrose, A. (2001). *Roland Penrose: The friendly surrealist*. National Galleries of Scotland.

Penrose, R. (n.d.). *Letter to Pailthorpe*. Unpublished manuscript. Scottish National Gallery of Modern Art, A62/1/108.

Polizzotti, M. (1995). *Revolution of the mind: The life of André Breton*. Farrar, Straus and Giroux.

Pollins, H. (1982). *Economic history of the Jews in Britain*. Associated University Presses.

Portman Clinic. (2008). The Portman Clinic: A historical note. Unpublished.

Rabaté, J. M. (2002). Loving Freud madly: Surrealism between hysterical and paranoid modernism. *Journal of Modern Literature*, *25*(3), 58–74.

Rank, O. (1924). *The trauma of birth*. Routledge, 2020.

Ray, P. (1971). *The surrealist movement in England*. Cornell University Press.

Read, H. (n.d.). *Correspondences*. Unpublished manuscript. Scottish National Gallery of Modern Art, RPA/718.

Read, H. (1934). From the first stroke. *The Listener*, *6*, 693–694.

Read, H. (1935, June 19). Writing into pattern: A new way of teaching art to children. *The Listener*, *13*, 1035–1036

Read, H. (1937–40). *Correspondences on Surrealism in Britain*. Unpublished manuscript. Scottish National Gallery of Modern Art, A62/1/101.

Read, H. (1938, January 26). The art of children. *The Listener*, *19*, 180.

Read, H. (1939). Bulletin mensuel de la FIARI. *Clé*, *I*, 4–5.

Read, H. (1939). L' Artiste dans le monde moderne. *Clé*, *II*, 7.

Read, H. (1940). *Correspondences on the Stafford Gallery exhibition*. Unpublished manuscript. Scottish National Gallery of Modern Art, A62/1/112.

Read, H. (1940). *Letter to Frank Norton*. Unpublished manuscript. Scottish National Gallery of Modern Art, A62/1/003.

Read, H. (1940). *Letters to Mednikoff on the Barcelona meeting*. Unpublished manuscript. Scottish National Gallery of Modern Art, A62/1/108.

Read, H., O'Brien, J., & Warren, R. P. (1939). The present state of poetry: a symposium: in England, in France, in the United States. *Kenyon Review*, *1*(4), 359–398.

Remy, M. (1986). *Surrealism in Britain in the thirties: Angels of anarchy and machines for making clouds [Exhibition catalog].* Leeds City Art Gallery.

Remy, M. (1999). *Surrealism in Britain.* Ashgate Publishing Company.

Rosemont, P. (1998). *Surrealist women: An international anthology.* University of Texas Press.

Ruszczynski, S. (2016). A brief introduction to the history of the Portman Clinic. *Journal of Child Psychotherapy, 3,* 262–265.

Rycroft, C. (1975). Dreams and the literary imagination. *The innocence of dreams* (pp. 153–167). Pantheon Books, 1979.

Sarner, M. (2022). A ninety-year history of the Portman Clinic. *International Journal of Forensic Psychotherapy, 4,* 12–20.

Saville, E., & Rumney, D. (1992). *A history of the I.S.T.D: A study of crime and delinquency from 1931 to 1992.* Institute for the Study and Treatment of Delinquency.

Sheehan-Dare, H. (1971). Dr. Grace W. *Pailthorpe. The President's New Bulletin, 24,* 26.

Short, R. (1978). *Surrealism unlimited.* Camden Art Centre.

Silber, E. (1986). *The sculpture of Epstein.* Phaidon.

Silberer, J. (1909). Report on a method of eliciting and observing certain symbolic hallucination-phenomena. In D. Rapaport (Ed.), *Organization and pathology of thought: Selected sources* (pp. 195–207). Columbia University Press, 1951.

Spalding, F. (2002). *British art since 1900.* Thames & Hudson.

Soothill, K., Peelo, M., & Taylor, C. (2002). *Making sense of criminology.* Polity.

Soupault, P. (1967, 1 April). *Souvenirs.* Nouvelle Revue Française, pp. 664–665.

Soupault, P. (1968). Origines et début du Surréalisme. *Europe,* n. 475–476 (November–December), pp. 3–6.

Soupault, P. (1980). *Vingt mille et un jours (Entretiens avec Serge Fauchereau).* Belfond.

Stefana, A. (2011). Introduzione al pensiero di Marion Milner. *Psicoterapia e Scienze Umane, 45*(3), 355–374.

Stefana, A. (2018). From *Die Traumdeutung* to The squiggle game: A brief history of an evolution. *American Journal of Psychoanalysis, 78,* 182–194.

Stefana, A. (2019). Revisiting Marion Milner's work on creativity and art. *International Journal of Psychoanalysis, 99,* 128–147.

Stefana, A. (2023). A brief introduction to Marion Milner's work on creativity and art. In M. Boyle Spelman & J. Raphael-Leff (Eds.), *The Marion Milner tradition* (pp. 125–133). Routledge.

Stefana, A., & Gamba, A. (2016). On the listening to the dreams of children affected by serious physical illness. *Minerva Pediatrica, 68*(1), 74–75.

Stefana, A., & Gamba, A. (2018). From the "squiggle game" to "games of reciprocity" towards a creative co-construction of a space for working with adolescents. *International Journal of Psychoanalysis, 99*(2), 355–379.

Stefana, A., & Gamba, A. (2023). *Marion Milner: A contemporary introduction.* Routledge.

Stefana, A., & Montanaro, L. A. (2023). *Introduction. In Grace Pailthorpe's writings on psychoanalysis and Surrealism.* Routledge.

Story, A. (1940). Correspondences on the Stafford Gallery exhibition. Unpublished *manuscript.* Scottish National Gallery of Modern Art, A62/1/112.

Swan, W. (2008). C.G. Jung's psychotherapeutic technique of active imagination in historical context. *Psychoanalysis and History, 10,* 185–204.

Thomas, G. (1943). Deflection of energy, as a result of birth trauma, and its bearing upon character formation: Grace W. Pailthorpe. *Psychoanalytic Quarterly, 12,* 593–593.

Topping, C. W. (1938). The report of the Royal commission on the penal system of Canada. *Canadian Journal of Economics and Political Science/Revue canadienne de economiques et science politique, 4*(4), 551–559.

Van der Hart, C., Omno, & Friedman, B. (1989). A reader's guide to Pierre Janet: A neglected intellectual heritage. *Dissociation, 2*(2).

Various authors. (1940). *London Bulletin, Nos. 18–20.* London Gallery Ltd.

Walker, J. (1944, June 14). Can't be ignored Surrealism has meaning to city artists. *The Province.*

Walker, J. (1974, June 14). Can't be ignored, Surrealism has meaning to city artists. *The Province.*

Walsh, N., & Wilson, A. (Eds.). (1998). *See sluice gates of the mind: The collaborative work of Pailthorpe and Mednikoff.* City Art Gallery.

Wolf, H. (2019). *A tale of mother's bones.* Camden Arts Centre.

Zemans, J. (1981). *Jock Macdonald: The inner landscape: A retrospective exhibition.* Art Gallery of Toronto.

Zemans, J. (2016). *Jock Macdonald: Life & work.* Art Canada Institute.

Index

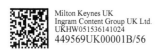